Register N~~ow~~
to

MW01484363

SPRINGER PUBLISHING
CⓊNNECT™

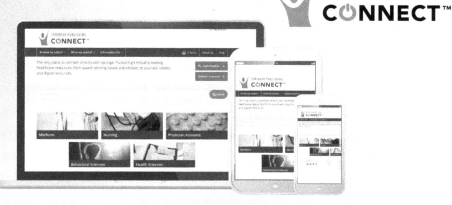

Your print purchase of *Telemental Health and Distance Counseling: A Counselor's Guide to Decisions, Resources, and Practice* **includes online access to the contents of your book**—increasing accessibility, portability, and searchability!

Access today at:
http://connect.springerpub.com/content/book/978-0-8261-7995-1 or scan the QR code at the right with your smartphone and enter the access code below.

3WGPT0C1

Scan here for quick access.

If you are experiencing problems accessing the digital component of this product, please contact our customer service department at cs@springerpub.com

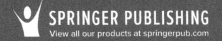

SPRINGER PUBLISHING
View all our products at springerpub.com

Heather C. Robertson, PhD, LMHC, LPC, CASAC, CRC, NCC, ACS, BC-TMH, is an Associate Professor of Counselor Education at St. John's University located in Jamaica, New York. She is the program coordinator for the Clinical Mental Health Counseling Program in the School of Education. She is a Licensed Professional Counselor (LPC, CT), Licensed Mental Health Counselor (LMHC, NY), Nationally Certified Counselor (NCC), Certified Rehabilitation Counselor (CRC), Credentialed Alcoholism and Substance Abuse Counselor (CASAC, NY), Approved Clinical Supervisor (ACS), Global Career Development Facilitator (GCDF), and Board Certified Telemental Health Provider (BC-TMH).

As BC-TMH and a former Distance Credentialed Counselor (DCC), Dr. Robertson's areas of research include telemental health counselor competence and distance counseling practices. She was awarded a 2018 North Atlantic Region Association for Counselor Education and Supervision research grant for her research entitled "Practice and Instruction of Distance Counseling: Educator, Supervisor, and Counselor Perspectives," and the 2020 Association for Counselor Education and Supervision research grant for her research entitled "Technological Training Interventions to Increase Counselor Competence." Her research has been presented at national and regional conferences on the topic of telemental health, specifically examining the preparation of professional counselors, counseling supervisors, and counselor educators.

Dr. Robertson's research and advocacy efforts include telemental health counselor preparation, substance abuse, military and veterans, career transition, and reducing the stigma of mental illness and addiction. She earned a PhD in Counselor Education and Supervision from Virginia Tech, an MS in Counseling and Guidance from Texas A & M University at Corpus Christi, and a bachelor's degree in Policy Studies from Syracuse University. Dr. Robertson served previously as the president of the American Counseling Association of New York (ACA-NY) and of the New York State Career Development Association.

Telemental Health and Distance Counseling

A Counselor's Guide to Decisions, Resources, and Practice

Heather C. Robertson, PhD, LMHC, LPC, CASAC, CRC, NCC, ACS, BC-TMH

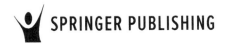 SPRINGER PUBLISHING

Springer Publishing Company, LLC
11 West 42nd Street, New York, NY 10036
www.springerpub.com
connect.springerpub.com/

Acquisitions Editor: Rhonda Dearborn
Compositor: Exeter Premedia Services Private Ltd.

ISBN: 978-0-8261-7994-4
ebook ISBN: 978-0-8261-7995-1
DOI: 10.1891/9780826179951

20 21 22 23 24 / 5 4 3 2 1

The author and the publisher of this Work have made every effort to use sources believed to be reliable to provide information that is accurate and compatible with the standards generally accepted at the time of publication. The author and publisher shall not be liable for any special, consequential, or exemplary damages resulting, in whole or in part, from the readers' use of, or reliance on, the information contained in this book. The publisher has no responsibility for the persistence or accuracy of URLs for external or third-party Internet websites referred to in this publication and does not guarantee that any content on such websites is, or will remain, accurate or appropriate.

LCCN: 2020946098

Contact sales@springerpub.com to receive discount rates on bulk purchases.

Publisher's Note: New and used products purchased from third-party sellers are not guaranteed for quality, authenticity, or access to any included digital components.

Printed in the United States of America.

This book is dedicated to the countless individuals who served on the front lines of the COVID-19 crisis, including medical workers, first responders, grocery workers, delivery drivers, postal carriers, stocking clerks, sanitation workers, and others. Thank you for putting your lives at risk for the protection of our safety. When you need support for your own mental health and emotion wellness, I hope you will allow the counseling profession to serve you, as you have served us during these challenging times.

Contents

Preface

The world changed dramatically between the start of this writing project in June of 2019, and the completion in June of 2020. My passion for research and writing this book emerged from a lingering concern that distance counseling (DC) and telemental health (TMH) were growing perhaps faster than counselors were being trained. My original proposal to Springer Publishing posited that counselors should pause, reflect, and carefully weigh any decisions before embarking on a DC/TMH practice. Counselors should determine the pros and cons of DC, and determine if TMH suits their practice before making the leap to providing distance services. What I could not have predicted in June of 2019 was how drastically the world would change by March of 2020 with the COVID-19 crisis and stay-at-home orders. Suddenly there was no choice; TMH and DC were the only option for professional counselors. That being said, even with the swift and abrupt transition to DC, my position has not changed—much. The earlier chapters in this book have been edited to reflect the reality of post-pandemic counseling, and later chapters fully include content pertaining to the COVID-19 crisis. You will note these eras being referred to as "pre-COVID-19" and "post-COVID-19," referencing the time frames before the onset of the pandemic and following it's emergence. For myself in New York, the onset and peak of the pandemic was March and April of 2020. For other regions, the onset and peak may vary.

This book is designed for professional counselors beginning their journey in DC, or continuing their practice of TMH. It is written for those who have been forced to practice via DC, as well as those who cannot decide if they want to engage in TMH practice. Chapter 1 provides the historical and evidence-based foundations of TMH, while Chapter 2 provides an overview of DC and TMH terminology, settings, and platforms, as well as certifications and training standards. This book is written from the perspective of a professional counselor; that being said, Chapters 3 through 8 are framed around the Council on the Accreditation of Counseling and

Related Education Programs (CACREP, 2016) core areas, including: Professional Orientation and Ethics, Psychosocial and Multicultural Development, Individual Counseling, Group Counseling, Career Development, and Assessment and Research. These chapters specifically address the use of DC and TMH within these foundational areas. Chapters 9 through 11 review DC and TMH within the CACREP counseling specialty areas including School Counseling, Student Affairs Counseling, Mental Health Counseling, Addictions Counseling, Rehabilitation Counseling, and Marriage, Couple, and Family Counseling. Career Counseling is excluded as a specialty area, since it is included as a foundational practice. These chapters include relevant professional literature, a review of appropriate ethical codes, case studies, critical questions in deciding to practice, as well as personal accounts provided by professional counselors engaging in distance counseling or telemental health, entitled "Voices From the Field."

A few notes on the universal elements of Chapters 3 through 11. The reader will note that the professional literature pulls from a variety of professions, including counseling, psychology, psychiatry, social work, and occasionally medicine. I attempt to provide the evidence base for DC and TMH, but also point out when that evidence is weak. While there is ample literature and evidence to support the effectiveness of TMH, it should be noted that rarely is DC evaluated as superior to in-person practice. It has been repeatedly found to be as effective as in-person treatment, and certainly more effective than no treatment at all. Ethical codes are reviewed for all major professional counseling organizations, with a specific emphasis on elements of the codes that address DC and TMH practice.

Case studies provide fictional examples of professional counselors using TMH interventions. Each case study is followed by open-ended questions designed to invite discussion on the various cases. The reader will note that every case asks the same closing question, "Assuming good intent, what did the counselor do well?" The truth is that most professional counselors are well intentioned, and they are committed to serving their clients with excellence. However, the nuances of DC and TMH can create challenges for the most well-meaning counselors. These cases and questions are not designed to alarm or stump readers, but to promote consideration of multiple perspectives. There will not necessarily be "correct" answers to these questions, but an opportunity for reflection and dialogue surrounding how to best respond in the designated scenario. Similarly, the "Critical Questions in Deciding to Practice" will also have no easy answers. These questions are designed to be answered based on the reader's personal experiences and skill set. The goal is for counselors to consider elements of their own practice, and how DC and TMH may support or hinder that practice.

The "Voices From the Field" entries represent the lived experiences of both professional counselors and counselor-interns who engage in DC and TMH practice. Some of these counselors were engaging in TMH prior to the COVID-19 crisis, while others were forced to transition following the pandemic. Their narratives provide real-life work experiences on the pros and cons of DC, as well as the unique aspects of TMH practice. In some cases, their voices echo the content from the chapter, while others provide new information based on their individual experience or client base. These voices address a variety of counseling practices and specializations including, individual, group, career, assessment, school, mental health, rehabilitation, and others.

Finally, Chapter 12 addresses the future of DC and TMH practice. As the use of DC becomes more common, counselors will need to navigate the changing complexities of newer technologies. Mobile applications ("apps") and self-help tools will be more common. Similarly, the profession of counseling will need to examine its position on TMH training, including adoption of credentialing standards. Counselor education programs will need to explore curricular content on DC. Most important, the professional counselor deciding to embark on a DC or TMH practice will need to carefully examine their own skills, experiences, training, clients, and professional ethics, as they weigh the pros and cons of practice. Technology will continue to grow and change; however, the counselor's commitment to client well-being and safety will not. This book is designed to give professional counselors the information and guidance to make personal decisions on DC and TMH practice—both in the wake of this pandemic and for years to come.

Heather C. Robertson

Acknowledgments

I'd like to thank several individuals for their support throughout this process. First of all, I would like to express my gratitude to Rhonda Dearborn at Springer Publishing for this opportunity and recognizing the timely and urgent need for this book. I am grateful to both Rhonda and Mehak Massand, for their continual guidance throughout this process. It's been an absolute pleasure working with you both on this project.

I would also like to thank St. John's University, specifically the Dean of the School of Education, Dr. David Bell, and the chair of the Counselor Education department, Dr. Robert Eshenauer, for their continued support of this project, while I attempted to manage my other roles at the university. I'd like to express sincere gratitude to Ryan Lowell, and Anna Wilga graduate students in Clinical Mental Health Counseling, who completed many edits and reviews of these chapters, often with increased pressure and tight deadlines. I am also grateful to the many colleagues and students who volunteered to provide their "Voices From the Field" experience for this book.

My family continues to support every endeavor I foolheartedly embark on. Thanks to my sisters, Michelle and Dana, for listening to me talk about "the book" on so many family Zoom meetings during quarantine. My mom, Lucille Sorrentino, might have missed her calling as editor-extraordinaire. At a certain age (I won't say what age), mom mastered online editing, simply to provide me with valuable and timely feedback on my writing. Finally, to my husband, Ben, and my boys, Ryan and Samuel. Thanks for enduring being quarantined with me, but never actually seeing me over the past few months while I finished this project. Your love and support drives everything I do.

1

History, Efficacy, and Demand for Telemental Health Counseling

INTRODUCTION

The profession of counseling is constantly evolving. From our foundational forces in psychoanalytic, humanistic, and behavioral therapy, multicultural and social justice forces have emerged. These fourth and fifth forces allow us to address the needs of our clients and students more equitably and effectively. With these changes in foundational forces, counseling theories have also evolved. This includes the emergence of post-modern and constructivist theories, as well as holistic and integrated theories, aimed at treating the person as a whole. Newer interventions, such as dialectical behavior therapy (DBT) and eye movement desensitization and reprocessing (EMDR) interventions have been developed to assist those with specific clinical needs. Thus it is little wonder that the format in which we practice counseling has also evolved. No longer confined to the couch of psychoanalysis, counseling interventions take place in schools, homes, and community settings, as well as online and in distance formats. Distance counseling (DC) and telemental health (TMH) may be considered two of the newest evolutions of the counseling profession, yet these practices have been in place for decades. This evolution to DC/TMH practice has been significantly hastened in a post-COVID-19 era, which required residents of 45 U.S. states to shelter-in-place (Mershov et al., 2020) forcing the majority of counseling services to a distance format.

The National Board of Certified Counselors (NBCC) was one of the first professional counseling organizations to publish standards for what was called at that time "web counseling" (NBCC, 1997, p. 3). Within those practice standards, web counseling was defined as "the practice of professional counseling and information delivery that occurs when client(s) and counselor are in separate or remote locations and utilize electronic means to communicate over the Internet" (NBCC, 1997, p. 3). While there have been many definitions of distance counseling and TMH, this early definition is a simple, longstanding representation of distance counseling. Specifically, the definition asserts that *professional counseling* is occurring. This distinction separates distance counseling from other distance practices, such as online information, self-help practices, or referral databases. The definition emphasizes using *electronic communication*. While electronic communication includes more than Internet services, this definition recognizes technology as the common denominator, which may include Internet, telephone, text, or other technological communication that evolves over time. While the client and counselor need not be in separate and remote locations for DC to occur (e.g., texting in the same room), the majority of distance sessions occur when clients and counselors are not in the same physical location.

DC and TMH have been referred to by many terms. In fact, Ostrowski and Collins' (2016) review of 65 state licensing boards' websites for counseling, psychology, and social work found 19 terms to describe TMH, including:

> distance counseling, distance therapy, electronic-assisted counseling, electronic means, electronic practice, electronic telepractice, electronic transmission, Internet counseling, Internet practice, online counseling, online psychotherapy, remotely, technology-assisted, teleconferencing, telehealth, telemental health, telepractice, telepsychology and teletherapy. (p. 390)

These findings demonstrate the struggle to both define and describe DC and TMH in a universal manner, despite the fact that professionals have been practicing TMH for over 50 years.

HISTORY OF TELEMEDICINE

The concept of offering counseling via distance modalities originally emerged in the field of medicine and was simultaneously adapted in the field of psychiatry. The earliest forms of telemedicine, now often referred to as e-health or telehealth, were used for unique medical conditions and to provide access to medical services in remote locations, such as rural communities, prisons, and combat regions. These were areas in which access to medical providers was scarce or impractical. Early use of telemedicine was designed to access specialized medical pathologists, while also eliminating the cost of transporting patients to medical providers (Breen & Matusitz, 2010). The first telemedicine study was conducted in Kansas in 1959 using a "two-way closed-circuit microwave television system" (Breen & Matusitz, 2010, p. 61), specifically to address patients' psychiatric needs. Around the same time, the National Aeronautics and Space Administration (NASA) began using telemedicine to assess astronauts' physical and emotional wellness. The American Psychiatric Association (APA) reports that, in 1969, psychiatrists from Massachusetts General Hospital provided telepsychiatry consultation to patients located at a clinic at Logan Airport. By the mid-1980s, telepsychiatry expanded to most therapeutic interactions, with telepsychiatry research and practice expanding globally into the 1990s (APA, n.d.).

The Samaritans established the first telephone counseling line for suicide prevention in London in 1953, which expanded to the United States in the early 1970s (Hornblow, 1986). These telephone services spread widely based on their "noninstitutional and generally nonprofessional orientation, their easy accessibility, and guaranteed anonymity" (Hornblow, 1986, p. 732). Use of telephone counseling increased based on public awareness, increased demand for psychological services, and efforts to connect people to help as soon as possible during periods of crisis (Hornblow, 1986).

The emergence of practice guidelines, such as those published by the American Telemedicine Association, solidified the dissemination of effective telepsychiatry practices (APA, n.d.). Practice guidelines were developed among other helping professions throughout the 1990s and 2000s. Specifically some of the earliest practice guidelines included:

- BCC, Standards for the Ethical Practice of WebCounseling (1997)
- Association of Social Work Boards (ASWB), Standards for Technology and Social Work Practice (2005)
- American Telemedicine Association (ATA), Core Operational Guidelines for Telehealth Services (2007)
- American Psychology Association (APA), Guidelines for the Practice of Telepsychology (2013)

While these guidelines have been updated and expanded over the years, they represent the first ethical and practical codes aimed specifically at the practice of counseling via distance modalities. The publication of these practice guidelines helped solidify distance counseling as an acceptable practice, recognized by leading professional organizations. The published standards and recognition lent credibility to its ethical utility in a counseling setting.

Information and communication technology improved greatly during the 2000s. Access to high quality video recording, audio recording, and transmission devices became widely available via Internet platforms. The emergence of video conferencing platforms, such as Skype™ and FaceTime™, provided reliable and often free access to videoconferencing technology. These technologies initially lacked confidentiality, encryption, and security. However newer platforms emerged that combined videoconferencing software with other technologies, such as instant messaging or email, and included encryption. These platforms could be purchased to provide TMH services within an organization or independently. Over the last decade, full turnkey platforms, such as Better Help™ and Talkspace™, have emerged integrating video, email, chat, and audio, as well as scheduling features. Within these platforms, a clinician joins a network of providers and becomes accessible to a wide variety of clients whom they are licensed to serve. These platforms are designed to be self-contained communication portals, which regularly build in encryption features to enhance security.

The growth of mobile applications, also known as "apps," has recently permeated the mental health market. In addition to counselor-facilitated technology, such as phone, email, videoconferencing, or messaging, a variety of automated and self-guided mental health tools have arrived on the market via apps. These tools allow clients and students to access mental health screenings, self-assessments, instructional coping techniques, and mechanisms to practice clinical treatments. While the use of apps by a client or student is not included in standard definitions of TMH or distance counseling, these apps are being used independently, or to supplement in-person or TMH counseling. The growth of the mobile app market demonstrates the acceptability of technology-assisted mental health practices, as well as the increased desire for on-demand services.

DEMAND FOR DISTANCE COUNSELING AND TELEMENTAL HEALTH

DC and TMH are more than phases or passing trends. In the wake of COVID-19, DC/TMH platforms became the norm, as opposed to the exception, yet even before the pandemic, TMH filled a treatment need in society. There is a shortage of mental health service providers in the United States. As of August 2019, the Health Resources and Services Administration (HRSA) indicated that there were 6,137 Health Professional Shortage Areas (HPSA) nationwide with a need for mental health services.

The highest mental health HPSAs were California, Texas, Michigan, and Arizona, yet mental health HPSAs were identified in nearly every state, as well as Puerto Rico (HRSA, 2019). TMH addresses these shortages by providing mental health services in areas that lack providers. Extensive literature supports the need for TMH, specifically to serve those in rural communities, veterans and military service members, individuals with access limitations, and those unlikely to access treatment.

Rural Communities

Traditional counseling in rural communities presents a number of challenges for both practitioners and clients. Traditional face-to-face (F2F) counseling requires clients to have access to mental health providers that are qualified, competent, and available to provide services. Due to low population density in rural areas, there are fewer mental health professionals available than required to meet the needs of the population (HRSA, 2019). Those mental health providers that are available often have full caseloads and a limited ability to expand services for a variety of reasons (Imig, 2014). First, if mental health providers are available, they may not specialize in a particular clinical issue or population needed by the client. For example, they may not have experience with the client's clinical need or diagnosis. They may not speak the language of the client, or may not belong to a particular cultural group that the client desires. Second, even when mental health counselors are available to provide counseling services, the issue of access to these services creates a challenge. In rural areas, practitioners and clients may be located many miles apart (Imig, 2014). Visiting a counselor in a traditional F2F setting can present excessive time and transportation costs for the client. These visits can significantly interrupt the client's regular weekly schedule in order to travel to and from a counseling appointment. In a F2F format, clients must have access to reliable transportation, most often a vehicle, as public transportation in rural communities may be sporadic or nonexistent. The burden is greater if the client receives services multiple times per week. Last, rural communities with low populations can create boundary issues for clients and counselors. Counselors and clients in smaller communities are more likely to know the same people, interact in similar settings, or utilize services from one another, simply due to the nature of small communities. These close connections create more opportunities for boundary crossings, by both the client and the counselor (Remley & Herlihy, 2016). Issues such as self-disclosure, breaches of confidentiality, or social interactions can unintentionally arise when serving as a lone practitioner in a close-knit rural community.

Distance counseling addresses these challenges by allowing clients the option to select a counselor that suits both their clinical and cultural needs, regardless of geographic location. As long as the selected TMH provider is licensed to serve the client, the client has more options in selecting a counselor. Clients seeking counselors with expertise in clinical foci, languages, or cultural characteristics have access to a wider range of counselor options with distance modalities. These options empower clients to select a counselor who meets their needs. The power to select their own provider outside of their geographic region also addresses the potential pitfalls of boundary-crossing among clients and counselors in small communities. TMH allows clients to access counseling services from a private, secure location that does not require travel beyond accessing their computer, mobile device, or phone. Immediate access reduces logistical costs for the client in the form of monetary travel costs, travel time, and interruption of their weekly activities. For clients needing more frequent sessions, these logistical costs would not increase. Data demonstrate that rural communities are increasing TMH utilization (Mehrotra et al., 2017), and counselors are providing TMH services from university medical centers, acute care hospitals, private providers, and rural health centers (Lambert et al., 2016, p. 371). In a study of rural women veterans who had experienced military sexual trauma (MST), clients saved an average of 172 miles per visit by receiving TMH services (Weiss et al., 2018).

Military Personnel and Veterans

U.S. military personnel serve their country from every corner of the globe. In addition to the geographic distance, military personnel are stationed in regions that are hostile and dangerous. While serving in these locations, military personnel witness violence, trauma, and loss. Military personnel face other stressors including separation from family, and, like their civilian counterparts, challenges with mental health and substance use. Being stationed abroad or deployed complicates access to mental healthcare. While mental health providers are available, the volume of trauma experienced can outweigh the coping strategies of the individual (Applewhite et al., 2012). In addition, military personnel may hesitate to seek mental health services, fearing that the stigma of mental illness will impact their ability to serve (Pargament & Sweeny, 2011). There is also evidence that some military personnel do not persist in mental health treatment (Harpaz-Rotem & Rosenheck, 2011).

The need for mental health services does not cease once the military member leaves service. The media has recently highlighted a variety of struggles that veterans in the United States face, including Posttraumatic Stress Disorder (PTSD), substance use, and suicide. The Department of Veterans Affairs (VA), which serves as the primary medical provider for veterans post-service, has been criticized for the excessive delays and limited capacity to serve the mental health needs of veterans (Llorca & Caruso, 2014). Similar to services provided in the field and those in rural communities, the demand for mental health services simply exceeds the supply of F2F mental health providers in VA hospitals.

The Department of Defense (DOD) and the VA have embraced and utilized TMH for decades, perhaps due to these challenges. The VA, despite challenges with traditional F2F services, has led the way in integrating TMH into their practice, including online screening tools, mobile apps, and providing TMH services. The VA has implemented an extensive menu of both telehealth and telemental health services. Current services include polytrauma services integrating social/emotional support (VA, 2018). The VA reports plans to develop additional TMH services including services for addiction, bipolar disorder, and schizophrenia (VA Telehealth Fact Sheet, n.d.). Beyond these synchronous services, the VA website promotes a variety of online tools for various mental health conditions. These tools address general mental health, depression and anxiety, PTSD, and substance use (VA, 2015).

Research supports the efficacy of TMH with military and veteran populations. A study comparing military members' and veterans' F2F treatment group to a TMH treatment group found both groups had a reduction in depressive symptoms; however, the F2F group experienced a more pronounced decrease in symptoms (Luxton et al., 2016). Acierno et al. (2016) examined two groups of veterans receiving treatment for PTSD, including a F2F group and TMH group. While both groups experienced a reduction in symptoms, the TMH group outcomes were not inferior to the F2F group outcomes (Acierno et al., 2016). Neither of these studies promote TMH as the superior service, yet both studies indicate a reduction of symptoms following TMH treatment. Due to the shortage of mental health providers, TMH provides an opportunity to serve military and veteran clients, while safely and effectively reducing symptoms.

Access Limitations

Individuals with access limitations may include those who have physical disabilities, individuals who are ill or elderly, those who do not have access to transportation, or those whose mental health condition limits their ability to interact with the outside community. Similar to those in rural communities, individuals with physical disabilities incur significant logistical costs to attend F2F counseling, including possibly the cost of a van service or use of an adaptive vehicle. In addition to the cost of transportation, individuals who use a wheelchair for mobility or another assistive mobility device need to concern themselves with accessible entryways and parking upon visiting a counselor's office. Individuals who are ill or elderly also need to address issues such as transportation, handrails, and stamina to travel to and from the counseling setting. Other studies demonstrate that lack of access for persons with disabilities may impact overall emotional well-being (Snook & Oliver, 2015). Lack of transportation, even in urban and suburban areas, can present an obstacle for individuals with mobility limitations that seek counseling (Bishop et al., 2013).

Individuals whose mental health condition limits their ability to interact with the community also struggle to attend traditional counseling sessions. These may include individuals with social anxiety, agoraphobia, and paranoid and/or delusional disorders (Dryman et al., 2017). School-aged students being home-schooled for medical and/or behavioral reasons may lack access to school counselors. Like veterans and those in rural communities, these groups benefit from TMH counseling in multiple ways. Some of these benefits include meeting in safe and secure locations, identifying specialists, connecting culturally to their counselor, and minimizing the costs, risks, or fears associated with travel.

Unlikely to Access Treatment

There is a growing body of literature suggesting that individuals who would not otherwise seek counseling services are utilizing DC and TMH. There is significant stigma surrounding mental health conditions, such as mental illness and substance use disorders. Many people fear that accessing a counselor via F2F methods may expose their potential mental health condition, making them vulnerable or susceptible to ridicule, judgment, or other negative factors (Pruitt et al., 2014). This fear of stigma has been well documented in military personnel (Pargament & Sweeny, 2011), as well as men (Masho & Alvanzo, 2010). Counseling may not be accepted in some cultures or families (Avent Harris et al., 2020). Individuals from these communities may hesitate to seek F2F counseling due to the stigma of discussing personal problems outside of the family or the church (Neely-Fairbanks et al., 2018). The emergence and success of crisis text lines demonstrate how text and type have become preferred communication mechanisms for some groups (Predmore et al., 2017). All of these groups benefit from the perceived anonymity of distance and TMH practices. While distance and TMH practices are not truly anonymous, the perception is that without being in the physical presence of another person, these individuals are more likely to communicate openly, without fear of ridicule and judgment that is so often associated with F2F counseling.

EFFICACY OF DISTANCE COUNSELING AND TELEMENTAL HEALTH

TMH counseling fills a need for a variety of populations, yet practitioners may question its effectiveness as a counseling modality. Research has demonstrated TMH to be as effective as traditional counseling services for multiple populations and conditions. DC has been utilized with adults, children, adolescents, parents, and the elderly. TMH has been utilized for a variety of mental health conditions including depression, anxiety, PTSD, attention deficit hyperactivity disorder (ADHD), eating disorders, substance use, as well as schizophrenia spectrum disorders.

Populations

Distance counseling has been utilized effectively with a wide variety of populations beyond those discussed. TMH has been used effectively with children and adolescents for issues such as ADHD, medication management, disruptive behavior disorders, and parent–child training programs (Comer et al., 2017; McCarty et al., 2015). In these studies, implementing services via video conferencing produced outcomes that were comparable or better to those receiving F2F treatments, with high satisfaction among TMH recipients. For children and adolescents, TMH services are provided in the home, as well as school settings, potentially reducing the stigma associated with attending mental health clinics (Nelson & Bui, 2010; Stephan et al., 2016).

Some counselors express concern that older adults will not respond to distance counseling or technology-enhanced services. Yet there is evidence that older adults are as responsive to TMH treatment and rate TMH health services favorably (Sheeran, Dealy, & Rabinowitz, 2013). Parents have also benefited from distance counseling and TMH interventions. Researchers have used TMH with couples counseling (Cicila et al., 2014), after pregnancy loss (Kersting et al., 2011), and with post-partum depression (Pugh et al., 2014), as well as with anxiety and depression during pregnancy (Loughnan et al., 2019).

Clinical Issues

A wide variety of clinical issues have been successfully treated with TMH, particularly utilizing cognitive behavioral therapy (CBT). TMH has been used successfully in populations with diagnoses of depression, anxiety, PTSD, substance use, smoking cessation, eating disorders, obsessive compulsive disorder, and insomnia, among others. Several studies using CBT TMH interventions for depression and anxiety have resulted in a reduction in symptoms, both at treatment completion and at post-intervention follow-up (Andersson et al., 2013; El Alaoui et al., 2016; Kivi et al., 2014; Moritz et al., 2012; Titov et al., 2010). TMH and CBT have been used with adults to address issues such as anxiety, depression (Hobbs et al., 2017), and psychiatric disorders (Mewton et al., 2013). Similarly, PTSD has been treated effectively using TMH interventions with college women (Littleton et al., 2016), victims of war and human rights violations, and veterans (Acierno et al., 2016; Yuen et al., 2015).

These studies represent only a fraction of the professional literature outlining the efficacy of TMH and DC. Hundreds of professional peer-reviewed articles have been published across the professions of psychiatry, psychology, social work, and professional counseling providing evidence of both the demand and effectiveness of TMH interventions. Few studies argue that TMH is more effective than F2F treatment, although many ascertain that additional research is needed to demonstrate its full effect. The majority of research supports TMH to be as effective as F2F treatment. In addition, studies find that TMH reduces symptoms for those not currently engaging in treatment, or can be used to augment F2F treatment. There is little evidence to demonstrate that TMH is ineffective with specific populations, such as those with more significant mental health disorders or those in crisis. The success of crisis text lines and hotlines suggests that TMH interventions are perhaps more effective, or at least more readily available in a crisis, than F2F interventions (Predmore et al., 2017).

DISTANCE COUNSELING ACROSS SPECIALIZATIONS

This book intentionally utilizes the term "distance counseling" along with TMH, such that individuals working both in and beyond mental health recognize how DC impacts their practice. Counselors in specialties other than mental health may feel disconnected from distance modalities based on the term "tele-MENTAL HEALTH," particularly if their scope of practice does not include mental health counseling. The majority of TMH research addresses mental health and substance use disorders. This is due to the fact that TMH emerged from telepsychiatry, as well as the increased attention on mental health shortages nationwide. Due to this focus, counselors may mistakenly assume that DC is reserved for those working in the mental health and substance use fields. This assumption would be both inaccurate and unwise, specifically as all counseling specialties transitioned to online modalities in the aftermath of the COVID-19 crisis. Multiple counseling specializations utilize DC, including school counseling, career counseling, clinical rehabilitation counseling, and others. The demand for DC described in this chapter applies to all counseling specializations, not strictly mental health. As evidence, consider the inclusion of technology in the recently published ethical codes of organizations such as the American School Counselors Association and the National Career Development Association.

Career counselors have utilized distance and online technologies for decades (Harris-Bowlsbey & Sampson, 2005; Mulcahy Boer, 2009), as computerized career guidance systems first emerged in the 1960s. Leading career development theorists have advocated for wider acceptance of online and distance practices among career practitioners (Bright, 2015; Kettunen et al., 2015), particularly with certain populations, such as college students (Venable, 2010). School counselors have also utilized distance technologies with students. A survey of nearly 800 school counselors revealed that 26% of school counselors utilized online technology to conduct remote individual and group counseling, psychoeducation, peer helping and consultation, while another 28% used online and remote technologies with students for advising and appraisal (Steele & Jacokes, 2015). Like career counselors, school counselors have advocated for more effective and ethical use of technology in the school counseling setting (Carlson et al., 2006; Wilczenski & Coomey, 2006). TMH is used effectively with students in a wide variety of school settings (Stephan et al., 2016).

All counselors, regardless of specialty, must now consider how distance modalities impact their counseling practice, including direct service, electronic communication, and record keeping. To disregard the impact of technology in these areas creates the risk of professional and ethical liability. While distance modalities impact all counseling specializations, not all counselors elect to engage in distance practices. This book aims to assist the counselor-reader in making an informed decision as to how you will use DC and TMH in your daily practice, if at all, regardless of your counseling setting. While the COVID-19 crisis thrust most counselors into TMH practice, this book emphasizes the counselor's decision. The choice to use TMH and DC lies with the provider, as well as the client/student.

LIMITATIONS

Numerous research studies support the demand for DC, and the effectiveness of TMH. Despite this evidence and support, there are potential obstacles and limitations with TMH delivery. While DC and TMH have the potential to provide greater access to counseling services for certain populations, individual access to TMH may be a limitation. Both the counselor and client must have access to the technology required to deliver TMH. Technology such as Internet bandwidth, Internet speed, landlines, mobile phone service, secure/encrypted phones, and Internet service is required to provide ethical and effective TMH services. These elements require financial means. They also require infrastructure to support these technologies. Issues such as power outages or poor service interrupt the quality of service provided. Thus TMH access is only as effective as the technology on which it's provided, and access to that technology requires financial resources. Limitations to accessing technology—which may include financial constraints of the individual or infrastructure constraints of a community—will impact delivery and utility of DC services.

State licensing laws also limit access. Laws on delivering TMH counseling differ from state to state, and change over time (Epstein Becker Green Law, 2020). Counselors need to be mindful of the legal statutes in their own state and their ability to deliver distance services to those in other locations. Insurance reimbursement for TMH, or lack thereof, will impact access as well. Different insurance providers have different policies on covering TMH and distance services. While many of these providers lifted restrictions during the COVID-19 crisis, these policies may place a financial burden on individuals seeking to use insurance for distance services or on the providers seeking to be reimbursed for TMH services. Providers also must be mindful to ensure that their liability insurance covers TMH delivery.

Confidentiality and security are potential limitations. In order to deliver TMH services, both client and counselor must have access to a secure and confidential setting to conduct sessions. Individuals in community residences or persons who lack privacy will struggle to safely and ethically utilize TMH. Counselors and clients must utilize proactive measures to protect privacy and ensure confidentiality, which may include encrypted devices, password protections, and security measures. Individuals who are unwilling or unable to engage in these additional security measures, or are unable to afford them, will be unable to safely and ethically engage in services.

Finally, while individuals may desire or demand distance counseling services, this modality may not be appropriate for all clients and counselors. Children and adolescents who are minors cannot utilize distance services without parent or guardian consent. Clients who lack the ability to use the required technology, either due to disability, developmental age, cognitive functioning, or access to technology, are not appropriate for TMH service delivery. Similarly, counselors who lack training and knowledge to appropriately utilize technology and conduct DC sessions cannot ethically and effectively provide services via distance modalities.

EDUCATION AND TRAINING DILEMMA

Counselors' hesitation to engage in DC may originate from lack of training. Counseling practitioners consistently express a desire for additional training in distance modalities (Baird et al., 2018; Centore & Milacci, 2008; Cipoletta & Mocellin, 2018; Perle et al., 2012; Simms et al., 2011). In the midst of the COVID-19 crisis, many counselors were given a "crash course" in TMH or simply dove in based on desire and/or directive to help. DC and TMH have not been consistently integrated into helping-profession graduate programs. Some professions, such as psychiatry and psychology, have actively advocated for the inclusion of TMH practices into curricula. Psychiatrists have advocated and effectively implemented TMH training in student training programs, embedding telepsychiatry into training and residency programs (Alicata et al., 2016; Glover et al., 2013; Hilty et al., 2015; Hoffman & Kane, 2013; Pullen et al., 2013; Sunderji et al., 2014). Psychologists have also advocated for inclusion of TMH within their professional training programs (Colbow, 2013). Counselors approach implementing DC in graduate-level training with caution. Researchers have successfully incorporated skill training for distance modalities, such as individual counseling (Haberstroh et al., 2008; Trepal et al., 2007) and group counseling (Kozlowski & Holmes, 2017) into counseling curricula.

Advocacy for DC training within graduate programs tends to focus on (a) adapting curricula to include TMH and DC, or (b) embedding training exercises into existing courses and curricula. Most traditional graduate-level training programs in the helping profession are guided by an accreditation process or standards established by a professional organization, such as the Council for the Accreditation of Counseling and Related Education Programs (CACREP) for counselor education programs. While these accrediting organizations are designed to be guidelines for training programs, graduate programs often utilize these guidelines to develop their training curriculum. Within these guidelines, there is no clear directive to train counselors to provide services via distance modalities. For example, CACREP requires accredited counselor education programs to address the *impact* of technology on the counseling process (CACREP, 2016, Section 2.F.1.j), but fails to require counselor education programs to provide training in TMH and DC. Thus, counselors from traditional training programs, including Clinical Mental Health, School, Career, Addictions, Rehabilitation, and others, may lack formal training in DC and TMH. Helping professions, such as psychology and social work, may face similar training shortfalls, although it is likely that these guidelines will change following the COVID-19 TMH transition.

Postgraduate training, or continuing education, is another training option to increase practitioner competence in DC and TMH. Anthony (2015) argues that postgraduate training (e.g., professional development training and/or certification) allows practitioners to learn the core skills of F2F counseling through their graduate program. Postgraduate training then allows those – who desire to learn about distance modalities – the option to specialize their skills in TMH. The challenge of postgraduate training appears to be varying requirements, credentials, and training content. In 2019, a Google search of the term "telemental health training" yielded 159,000 results in .55 seconds; "Distance counseling training" yielded 44.5 million on .59 seconds. "Distance counseling certification" yielded 12.3 million while "telemental health certification" yielded 39,000; "telemental health license" yielded 163,000 and "distance counseling license" produced 9.5 million results—each in less than one second. The amount of information available is vast and not necessarily reliable, leaving the clinician seeking postgraduate training with little guidance in the process. There are training programs that are valid, reputable, and endorsed by respected counseling and mental health organizations for the counselor who knows how to find them. However, these training programs lack a standard accreditation process to unify the training content and requirements.

Lack of unified training standards, varying training content, and multiple options for postgraduation credentials contribute to counseling practitioners' hesitancy to engage in DC or TMH practice. This book aims to provide objective and reliable information on DC practices, illuminate ethical issues, and identify resources that will guide practitioners in their decision whether or not to expand their practices via distance modalities.

CONCLUSION

The use of DC and TMH has been utilized in the helping professions for decades, prior to the significant increase following the COVID-19 outbreak. Telephone and video sessions have been in place since the 1950s and 1960s. As professional organizations developed TMH practice guidelines, the acceptance of DC/TMH interventions grew. Demand for these interventions are prevalent among rural communities, military personnel and veterans, those with access limitations, and those unlikely to seek treatment. More importantly, DC and TMH has been found to be effective for a wide variety of populations and clinical issues, as well as across counseling specializations. There are limits to distance counseling including licensure laws, technological access, issues with confidentiality and privacy, as well as training. Prior to COVID-19, professional counselors were not regularly trained in DC/TMH interventions, and many counselors reported a need for training in order to increase their confidence in practice. Lack of unified training standards contribute to confusion and uncertainty among counselors and clients alike.

REFERENCES

Acierno, R., Gros, D. F., Ruggiero, K. J., Hernandez-Tejada, B. M. A., Knapp, R. G., Lejuez, C. W., Muzzy, W., Frueh, C. B., Egede, L. E., & Tuerk, P. W. (2016). Behavioral activation and therapeutic exposure for post- traumatic stress disorder: A noninferiority trial of treatment delivered in-person versus home based telemental health. *Depression and Anxiety, 33*, 415–423. https://doi .org/10.1002/da.22476

Alicata, D., Schropher, A., Unten, T., Aghora, R., Helm, S., Fukada, M., Ulrich, D., & Michaels, S. (2016). Telemental health training, team building, and workforce development in cultural contexts: The Hawaii experience. *Journal of Child and Adolescent Psychopharmacology, 3*, 260–265. https://doi.org/10.1089/cap.2015.0036

American Psychiatric Association. (n.d.). *Telepsychiatry tool kit: History of telepsychiatry.* https://www.psychiatry.org/psychiatrists/practice/telepsychia try/toolkit/history-of-telepsychiatry

American Psychology Association. (2013). *Guidelines for the practice of telepsychology.* https://www.apa.org/pubs/journals/features/amp-a0035001.pdf

American Telemedicine Association. (2007). *Core operational guidelines for telehealth services.* https://www.americantelemed.org/resources/core-operational-guidelines-for-telehealth-services-involving-provider-patient-interactions/

Andersson, G., Hesser, H., Hummerdal, D., Bergman-Nordgren, L., & Carlbring, P. (2013). A 3.5-year follow-up of Internet-delivered cognitive behavior therapy for major depression. *Journal of Mental Health, 22*, 155–164. https://doi.org/10 .3109/09638237.2011.608747

Anthony, K. (2015). Training therapists to work effectively online and offline within digital culture. *British Journal of Guidance & Counselling, 43*(1), 36–42. https://doi.org/10.1080/03069885.2014.924617

Applewhite, L., Keller, N., & Borah, A. (2012). Mental health care use by soldiers conducting counterinsurgency operations. *Military Medicine, 177*, 501–506. https://doi.org/10.7205/MILMED-D-11-00142

Association of Social Work Boards. (2005). *Standards for technology and social work practice.* https://www.labswe.org/assets/Docs/NASW_ASWB_Stds_for_Tech _and_SW_Practice.pdf

Avent Harris, J. R., Crumb, L., Crowe, A., & Garland McKinney, J. (2020). African American's perceptions of mental illness and preferences for treatment. *Journal of Counselor Practice, 11*(1), 1–22. https://doi.org/10.22229/afa1112020

Baird, M. B., Whitney, L., & Caedo, C. E. (2018). Experiences and attitudes among psychiatric mental health advanced practice nurses in the use of telemental health: Results of an online survey. *Journal of the American Psychiatric Nurses Association, 24*(3), 235–240. https://doi.org/10.1177/1078390317717330

Bishop, M., Frain, M., Rossler, R. T., Waletich, B., Rumrill, P. D., Umeasigbu, V., & Sheppard-Jones, K. (2013). The relationship between housing variables and employment status among adults with multiple sclerosis. *Journal of Rehabilitation, 79*(4), 4–14.

Breen, G. M., & Matusitz, J. (2010). An evolutionary examination of telemedicine: A health and computer-mediated communication perspective. *Social Work Public Health,* 25(1): 59–71. https://doi.org/10.1080/19371910902911206

Bright, J. E. H. (2015). If you go down to the woods today, you are in for a big surprise: Seeing the wood for the trees in online delivery of career guidance. *British Journal of Guidance & Counselling, 43,* 24–35. https://doi.org/10.1080/03069885.2014.979760

Carlson, L. A., Portman, T. A. A., Bartlett, J. A. (2006). Professional school counselors' approaches to technology. *Professional School Counseling, 9,* 252–256. https://doi.org/10.5330/prsc.9.3.9162536405845454

Centore, A. J., & Milacci, A. (2008). A study of mental health counselor's use and perspectives on distance counseling. *Journal of Mental Health Counseling, 30,* 267–282. https://doi.org/10.17744/mehc.30.3.q871r684n863u75r

Cicila, L. N., Georgia, E. J., & Doss, B. D. (2014). Incorporating Internet-based Interventions into couple therapy: Available resources and recommended Uses. *Australian & New Zealand Journal of Family Therapy, 35*(4), 414–420. https://doi.org/10.1002/anzf.1077

Cipoletta, S., & Mocellin, D. (2018). Online counseling: An exploratory survey of Italian psychologists' attitudes toward new ways of interaction. *Psychotherapy Research, 28,* 909–924. https://doi.org/10.1080/10503307.2016.1259533

Colbow, A. J. (2013). Looking to the future: Integrating telemental health therapy into psychologist training. *Training and Education in Professional Psychology, 3,* 155–165. https://doi.org/10.1037/a0033454

Comer, J. S., Furr, J. M., Miguel, E. M., Cooper-Vince, C. E., Carpenter, A. L., Elkins, R. M., Kerns, C. E., Cornacchio, D., Chou, T., Coxe, S., DeSerisym M., Sanchez, A. L., . . . Chase, R. (2017). Remotely delivering real-time parent training in the home: An initial randomized trial of Internet-delivered Parent-Child Interaction Therapy (I-PCIT). *Journal of Consulting and Clinical Psychology, 85,* 909–917. https://doi.org/10.1037/ccp0000230

Council for the Accreditation of Counseling and Related Education Programs. (2016). *2016 CACREP standards.* https://www.cacrep.org/for-programs/2016-cacrep-standards/

Dryman, M. T., McTeague, L. M., Olino, T. M., & Heimberg, R. G. (2017). Evaluation of an open-access CBT-based internet program for social anxiety: Patterns of use, retention, and outcomes. *Journal of Consulting & Clinical Psychology, 85,* 988–1000. https://doi.org/10.1037/ccp0000232

El Alaoui, S., Ljótsson, B., Hedman, E., Svanborg, C., Kaldo, V., & Lindefors, N. (2016). Predicting outcome in Internet-Based Cognitive Behaviour Therapy for major depression: A large cohort study of adult patients in routine psychiatric care. *PLoS ONE, 11*(9), 1–16. https://doi.org/10.1371/journal.pone.0161191

Epstein Becker Green Law. (2020). *Telemental health laws update.* https://www.ebglaw.com/covid-19-telemental-health-laws-update/

Glover, J. A., Williams, E., Hazlett, L. J., & Campbell, N. (2013). Connecting to the future: Telepsychiatry in post graduate medical education. *Telemedicine and e-Health, 19,* 474–479. https://doi.org/10.1089/tmj.2012.0182

Haberstroh, S., Parr, G., Bradley, L., Morgan-Flemming, B., & Gee, R. (2008). Facilitating online counseling: Perspectives from counselors in training. *Journal of Counseling & Development, 86,* 460–470. https://doi.org/10.1002/j.1556-6678.2008.tb00534.x

Harpaz-Rotem, I., & Rosenheck, R. A. (2011). Serving those who served: Retention of newly returning veterans from Iraq and Afghanistan in mental health treatment. *Psychiatric Services, 62,* 22–27. https://doi.org/10.1176/ps.62.1.pss6201_0022

Harris-Bowlsbey, J., & Sampson. (2005). Use of technology in delivering career services worldwide. *The Career Development Quarterly, 54,* 48–56. https://doi.org/10.1002/j.2161-0045.2005.tb00140.x

Health Resources and Services Administration. (2019, August 16). *Shortage areas.* https://data.hrsa.gov/topics/health-workforce/shortage-areas

Hilty, D. M., Crawford, A., Teshima, J., Chan, S., Sunderji, N., Yellowlees, P. M., Kramer, G., O'neill, P., Fore, C., Luo, J., & Li, S. (2015). A framework for telepsychiatric training and e-health: Competency-based education, evaluation and implications. *International Review of Psychiatry, 27,* 569–592. https://doi.org/10.3109/09540261.2015.1091292

Hobbs, M. J., Mahoney, A. E. J., & Andrews, G. (2017). Integrating iCBT for generalized anxiety disorder into routine clinical care: Treatment effects across the adult lifespan. *Journal of Anxiety Disorders, 51,* 47–54. https://doi.org/10.1016/j.janxdis.2017.09.003

Hoffman, P., & Kane, J. M. (2013). Telepsychiatry education and curriculum development in residency training. *Academic Psychiatry, 39,* 108–109. https://doi.org/10.1007/s40596-013-0006-6

Hornblow, A. R. (1986). The evolution and effectiveness of telephone counseling services. *Hospital and Community Psychiatry, 37,* 731–733. https://doi.org/10.1176/ps.37.7.731

Imig, A. (2014). Small but mighty: Perspectives of rural mental health counselors. *The Professional Counselor, 4,* 404–412. https://doi.org/10.15241/aii.4.4.404

Kersting, A., Kroker, K., Schlicht, S., Baust, K., & Wagner, B. (2011). Efficacy of cognitive behavioral internet-based therapy in parents after the loss of a child during pregnancy: Pilot data from a randomized controlled trial. *Archives of Women's Mental Health, 14,* 465–477. https://doi.org/10.1007/s00737-011-0240-4

Kettunen, J., Sampson, J. P., & Vuourinen, R. (2015). Career practitioners' conceptions of competency for social media in career services. *British Journal of Guidance & Counseling, 43,* 43–56. https://doi.org/10.1080/03069885.2014.939945

Kivi, M., Eriksson, M. C. M., Hange, D., Petersson, E., Vernmark, K., Johansson, B., & Björkelund, C. (2014). Internet-based therapy for mild to moderate depression in Swedish primary care: Short term results from the PRIM-NET Randomized Controlled Trial. *Cognitive Behaviour Therapy, 43,* 289–298. https://doi.org/10.1080/16506073.2014.921834

Kozlowski, K. A., & Holmes, C. M. (2017). Teaching online group counseling skills in an on- campus group counseling course. *The Journal of Counselor Preparation and Supervision, 9*(1). https://doi.org/10.7729/91.1157

Lambert, D., Gale, J., Hartley, D., Croll, Z., & Hansen, A. (2016). Understanding the business case for telemental health in rural communities. *Journal of Behavioral Health Services & Research, 43,* 366–379. https://doi.org/10.1007/s11414-015-9490-7

Llorca, J. C., & Caruso, D. B. (2014, June 11). Long waits persist for vets seeking mental health care at VA medical centers. *US News and World Report/ Associated Press.* http://www.usnews.com/news/us/articles/2014/06/11/long-waits-at-the-va-for-mental-health-care

Littleton, H., Grills, A. E., Kline, K. D., Schoemann, A. M., & Dodd, J. C. (2016). The From Survivor to Thriver program: RCT of an online therapist-facilitated program for rape- related PTSD. *Journal of Anxiety Disorders, 43,* 41–52. https://doi.org/10.1016/j.janxdis.2016.07.010

Loughnan, S. A., Sie, A., Hobbs, M. J., Joubert, A. E., Smith, J., Haskelberg, H., Mahoney, A. E. J., Kladnitski, N., Holt, C. J., Milgrom, J., Austin, M-P., Andrews, G., & Newby, J. M. (2019). A randomized controlled trial of 'MUMentum Pregnancy': Internet-delivered cognitive behavioral therapy program for antenatal anxiety and depression. *Journal of Affective Disorders, 243,* 381–390. https://doi.org/10.1016/j.jad.2018.09.057

Luxton, D. D., Pruitt, L. D., Wagner, A., Smolenski, D. A., Jenkins-Guarnieri, M. A., & Gahm, G. (2016). Home-based telebehavioral health for U.S. military personnel and veterans with depression: A randomized controlled trial. *Journal of Consulting and Clinical Psychology, 84,* 923–934. https://doi.org/10.1037/ccp0000135

Masho, S. W., & Alvanzo, A. (2010). Help-seeking behavior among men sexual assault survivors. *American Journal of Men's Health, 4,* 237–242. https://doi.org/10.1177/1557988309336365

McCarty, C. A., Vander Stoep, A., Violette, H., & Myers, K. (2015). Interventions developed for psychiatric and behavioral treatment in the children's ADHD telemental health treatment study. *Journal of Child and Family Studies, 24,* 1735–1743. https://doi.org/10.1007/s10826-014-9977-5

Mehrotra, A., Huskamp, H. A., Souza, J., Uscher-Pines, L., Rose, S., Landon, B. E., Jena, A. B., & Busch, A. B. (2017). Rapid growth in mental health telemedicine use among rural Medicare beneficiaries, wide variation across states. *Health Affairs, 36,* 909–917. https://doi.org/10.1377/hlthaff.2016.1461

Mershov, S., Lu, D., & Swales, V. (2020, April 20). See which states and cities have told residents to stay home. *The New York Times.* https://www.nytimes.com/interactive/2020/us/coronavirus-stay-at-home-order.html

Mewton, L. , Sachdev, P. S., & Andrews, G. (2013). A naturalistic study of the acceptability and effectiveness of internet-delivered cognitive behavioural therapy for psychiatric disorders in older Australians. *PLoS ONE, 8*(8), 1–5. https://doi.org/10.1371/journal.pone.0071825

Moritz, S., Schilling, L., Hauschildt, M., Schröder, J., & Treszl, A. (2012). A randomized controlled trial of internet-based therapy in depression. *Behaviour Research & Therapy, 50,* 513–521. https://doi.org/10.1016/j.brat.2012.04.006

Mulcahy Boer, P. (2009). *Career counseling over the internet: An emerging model for trusting and responding to online clients.* Lawrence Erlbaum Associates Inc. Publishers.

National Board for Certified Counselors. (1997). Standards for the ethical practice of WebCounseling, *NBCC News Notes, 14*(2), 3–4. http://www.nbcc.org/Assets/Newsletter/Issues/fall97.pdf

Neely-Fairbanks, S. Y., Rojas-Guyler, L., Nabors, L., & Banjo, O. (2018). Mental illness knowledge, stigma, help-seeking behaviors, spirituality, and the African American church. *American Journal of Health Studies, 33,* 162–174. http://www.va-ajhs.com/33-4/index.aspx

Nelson, E., & Bui, T. (2010). Rural telepsychology services for children and adolescents. *Journal of Clinical Psychology: In Session, 66,* 490–501. https://doi.org/10.1002/jclp.20682

Ostrowski, J., & Collins, T. (2016). A comparison of telemental health terminology used across mental health state licensing boards. *The Professional Counselor, 6,* 387–396. https://doi.org/10.15241/jo.6.4.387

Pargament, K. I., & Sweeny, P. J. (2011). Building spiritual fitness in the Army: An innovative approach to a vital aspect of human development. *American Psychologist, 66,* 58–64. https://doi.org/10.1037/a0021657

Perle, J. G., Langsam, L. C., Randel, A., Lutchman, S., Levine, A. B., Odland, A. P., Nierenberg, B., & Marker, C. D. (2012). Attitudes toward psychological telehealth: Current and future clinical psychologists opinions of internet-based interventions. *Journal of Clinical Psychology, 69,* 100–113. https://doi.org/10.1002/jclp.21912

Pugh, N., Hadjistavropoulos, H., & Fuchs, C. (2014). Internet therapy for postpartum depression: A case illustration of emailed therapeutic assistance. *Archives of Women's Mental Health, 17,* 327–337. https://doi.org/10.1007/s00737-014-0439-2

Predmore, Z., Ramchand, R., Ayer, L., Kotzias, V., Engel, C., Ebener, P., Kemp, J. E., Karras, E., & Hass, G. L. (2017). Expanding suicide crisis services to text and chat. *Crisis, 38,* 255–260. https://doi.org/10.1027/0227-5910/a000460

Pruitt, L. D., Luxton, D. D., & Shore, P. (2014). Additional clinical benefits of home-based telemental health treatments. *Professional Psychology: Research and Practice, 45,* 340– 346. https://doi.org/10.1037/a0035461

Pullen, S. J., White, J. C., Salgado, C. A., Sengupta, S., Takala, C. R., Tai, S., Swintak, C., & Shatkin, J. P. (2013). Video-teleconferencing with medical students to improve exposure to child and adolescent psychiatry. *Academic Psychiatry, 34,* 268–270. https://doi.org/10.1176/appi.ap.12040073

Remley, T. P., & Herlihy, B. (2016). *Ethical, legal, and professional issues in counseling.* Pearson.

Sheeran, T., Dealy, J., & Rabinowitz, Y. (2013). Geriatric telemental health. In K. Myers & C. Turvey (Eds), *Telemental health: Clinical, technical, and administrative foundations for evidence-based practice.* Elsevier

Simms, D. C., Gibson, K., & O'Donnell, S. (2011). To use or not to use: Clinicians' perceptions of telemental health. *Canadian Psychology, 52,* 41–51. https://doi.org/10.1037/a0022275

Snook, J., & Oliver, M. (2015). Perceptions of wellness from adults with mobility impairments. *Journal of Counseling & Development, 93,* 289–297. https://doi .org/10.1002/jcad.12027

Steele, T. M., & Jacokes, D. E. (2015). An examination of the role of online technology in school counseling. *Professional School Counseling, 18,* 125–135. https://doi .org/10.5330/prsc.18.1.428818712j5k8677

Stephan, S., Lever, N., Bernstein, L., Edwards, S., & Pruitt, D. (2016). Telemental health in schools. *Journal of Child and Adolescent Psychopharmacology, 26,* 266–272. https://doi.org/10.1089/cap.2015.0019

Sunderji, N., Crawford, A., & Jovanovic, M. (2014). Telepsychiatry in graduate medical education: A narrative review. *Academic Psychiatry, 39,* 55–62. https:// doi.org/10.1007/s40596-014-0176-x

Titov, N., Andrews, G., Davies, M., McIntyre, K., Robinson, E., & Solley, K. (2010). Internet treatment for depression: A randomized controlled trial comparing clinician vs. technician assistance. *PLoS ONE, 5*(6), 1–9. https://doi.org/10.1371/ journal.pone.0010939

Trepal, H., Haberstroh, S., Duffey, T., & Evans, M. (2007). Considerations and strategies for teaching online counseling skills: Establishing relationships in cyberspace. *Counselor Education & Supervision, 46,* 266–279. https://doi .org/10.1002/j.1556-6978.2007.tb00031.x

Venable, M. (2010). Using technology to delivery career development services: Supporting today's students in higher education. *The Career Development Quarterly, 59,* 87–96. https://doi.org/10.1002/j.2161-0045.2010.tb00132.x

Veterans Affairs. (n.d.). *VA Telehealth services fact sheet.* https://www.va.gov/ COMMUNITYCARE/docs/news/VA_Telehealth_Services.pdf

Veterans Affairs. (2015). *Mental health self-help resources.* https://www.mentalhealth .va.gov/self_help.asp

Veterans Affairs. (2018). *VA telehealth services.* https://telehealth.va.gov/

Weiss, B. J., Azevedo, K., Webb, K., Gimeno, J., & Cloitre, M. (2018). Telemental health delivery of Skills Training in Affective and Interpersonal Regulation (STAIR) for rural women veterans who have experienced military sexual trauma. *Journal of Traumatic Stress, 31,* 620–625. https://doi.org/10.1002/jts.22305

Wilczenski, F. L., & Coomey, S. M. (2006). Cyber-communication: Finding its place in school counseling practice, education, and professional development. *Professional School Counseling, 9,* 327–331. https://doi.org/10.5330/prsc.9.4 .78t6014366615205

Yuen, E. K., Gros, D. F., Price, M. Ziegler, P., Tuerk. P. W., Foa, E. B., & Acierno, R. (2015). Randomized controlled trial of home-based telemental health versus prolonged exposure for combat related PTSD in veterans: Preliminary results. *Journal of Clinical Psychology, 7,* 500–513. https://doi.org/10.1002/jclp.22168

2

Overview of Distance Counseling and Telemental Health

INTRODUCTION

New experiences can be uncomfortable, even when someone has decided to pursue that new experience of their own free will. While distance counseling (DC) and telemental health (TMH) are not new, the practice of DC and TMH may be new to some counselors. Think back to your original coursework in counseling skills. There appeared to be so many new skills: attending, paraphrasing, probing, reflecting feeling, interpretation, observing non-verbal behaviors, including multicultural differences, and more. A student once said that learning counseling skills is like learning how to drive a car. She stated that when you first learn to drive a car, there are so many moving parts: checking mirrors, paying attention to traffic on all sides, observing street signs, using turn signals, watching your speed, and more. She said, "Initially it's overwhelming, but after a while, it becomes more natural, and you just drive." The manner in which we learn counseling skills is much the same: Initially it appears as if there are many moving parts, but after a while, it becomes more natural, you develop your personal style, and counsel. Distance counseling adds a new element to a familiar practice. Using the driving metaphor, it's as if you learned to drive on an automatic, but now you are being asked to drive a stick shift or a motorcycle. You know how to drive, but something is new, different, uncomfortable, and maybe even a bit frightening. DC and TMH are similar to learning that stick shift or motorcycle. We apply many of the same skills used in face-to-face (F2F) counseling, but there are new elements that require training, as well as caution. This chapter is designed to provide an overview of those elements, and to make this new and uncertain practice somewhat more familiar.

DEFINITIONS AND TERMINOLOGY

Understanding terms regularly utilized in DC and TMH is essential to understanding the practice. Selected key terms are described and defined in the following.

Distance Counseling

DC was first defined as a component of the Distance Credentialed Counselor (DCC) training program in 2003, developed by an organization called ReadyMinds (Malone, 2007). Through this training, DC "employs the thoughtful use of technologies (synchronous, asynchronous, and computerized counseling programs) in order to assist clients to function with, or grow towards, increased wellness in their personal and professional lives" (Malone, 2007, p. 3). In this book, the term DC is used collaboratively with TMH in order to include non-mental-health counseling specialties, such as school or career counseling.

Telemental Health

TMH is more difficult to define, since many definitions of TMH are derived from telehealth or telemedicine. A variety of definitions for TMH can be located on the Zur Institute's website (www .zurinstitute.com/telehealth-define/), which references definitions from organizations such as the American Psychological Association, American Telemedicine Association, and others. Luxton, Nelson, and Maheu (2016) succinctly define TMH as "the practice of either clinical or nonclinical aspects of healthcare provided via communications technology" (p. 9). It's important to note that Medicare has separate definitions and limitations on the provision of telemedicine (Luxton et al., 2016). In addition, definitions and guidelines for practicing TMH vary from state to state (Epstein Becker Green Law, 2020).

Health Insurance Portability and Accountability Act

The Health Insurance Portability and Accountability Act (HIPAA) was enacted in 1996,

> to improve portability and continuity of health insurance coverage in the group and individual markets, to combat waste, fraud, and abuse in health insurance and healthcare delivery, to promote the use of medical savings accounts, to improve access to long-term care services and coverage, to simplify the administration of health insurance, and for other purposes. (U.S. Department of Health and Human Services [DHHS], 1996, para. 1)

The HIPAA Privacy Rule, enacted in 2000, defined **protected health information (PHI)**. The Privacy Rule protects identifiable health information (or PHI) from being disclosed to any third party without authorization. In 2003, the enactment of the Security Rule designated that **electronic protected health information (ePHI)** stored in electronic medical record systems or transmitted electronically was also protected from disclosure without authorization (DHHS, 2017). Due to the digital nature of DC and TMH, following HIPAA guidelines is essential to ethical practice.

Synchronous

Synchronous services occur in real time, such as telephone conversations or video conferencing sessions. Synchronous services are considered "live" and involve the counselor and client being present concurrently. More specifically, synchronous services allow for communication to go in both directions, or multiple directions in the case of group counseling, at the same time (Myers & Turvey, 2013).

Asynchronous (Store and Forward)

Asynchronous services are considered the opposite of synchronous services. Communication goes in one direction at a time, such as email or text messages. These services are sometimes referred to as "store and forward" services that reference messages, emails, photos, or videos that are created and sent to the recipient. The recipient may receive these messages immediately, or may retrieve them at a later time (Myers & Turvey, 2013).

Encryption

According to the U.S. Department of Commerce's National Institute for Standards of Technology's (NIST) glossary of cyber security terms, encryption has several definitions. Specifically, the process of encryption changes plain text to cipher text, with the goal of preventing anyone but the intended party from receiving or interpreting the information. More clearly, encryption is defined as the "the process of a confidentiality mode that transforms usable data into an unusable form" (NIST, n.d., para. 9). TMH and DC utilize a variety of technological devices such as telephones, software, computers, and the Internet to communicate with their clients. Safety and confidentiality are key components of ethical counseling practice, warranting the need to utilize encrypted devices and systems.

These terms represent only a sample of the common terms used when discussing TMH and DC. Other terminology may be utilized and will be defined throughout this book, yet these common terms provide a foundation for discussion. Technological terms may be confusing or unclear to clients and students. It is the counselor's responsibility to explain services in a language that clients and students can understand.

SETTINGS

DC and TMH are practiced in various settings. For some counselors and clients, the use of TMH is intentional and deliberate—meaning that both the client and the counselor opted to utilize TMH for counseling. There are a multitude of reasons as to why one would intentionally select distance counseling beyond simply finding it "more convenient." Specifically, clients in rural communities, those who have travel or mobility limitations, as well as those who fear the stigma of seeking counseling are commonly served via distance counseling (Dryman et al., 2017; Mehrotra et al., 2017; Pruitt et al., 2014). In addition, clients who seek specialized providers, such as counselors with a particular clinical focus, language ability, or demographic, may elect to use TMH in order to access a wide range of counselors. Intentional TMH practice may utilize one or several modalities, including but not limited to telephone, video conferencing, email, or text/chat. When DC is intentional, the counselor establishes their distance practice using security features, encrypted technology, and a detailed informed consent. The counselor also screens clients for DC appropriateness via the selected modality.

DC also occurs in unplanned or unintentional settings. This may include crisis situations with F2F clients, or planned absences from traditional F2F sessions. In crisis situations, clients may contact counselors with a need for immediate support due to crisis. Counselors who agree to this emergency session may elect to conduct the unplanned session via a distance modality, such as phone, text, email, or other modality. Similarly, when a client or counselor is going to be absent during regularly scheduled sessions, counselors and clients may elect to conduct a session via distance modality. One of the challenges in these situations is that the client may not have been screened for DC appropriateness, and may not have been informed on the risks and requirements of DC. Thus, even when a counselor does not normally conduct sessions via DC, it helps to have a policy on emergency situations and absences in the informed consent document. If the counselor's policy allows distance sessions in these circumstances, guidelines should be established, such as using secure devices and code words, maintaining confidentiality and privacy, screening for appropriateness, and risks of conducting DC.

PLATFORMS

DC is conducted via synchronous, asynchronous, blended, and turnkey platforms. While these are current platforms used for DC, it is expected that variations on these platforms, if not entirely new platforms, will emerge in the future. As discussed, synchronous platforms allow counseling to be conducted in real time, meaning that the client(s) and counselor are both present and communicating in real time. The most commonly utilized synchronous platforms are telephone and videoconferencing. Some platforms such as instant messenger or chat may be considered live; however, these platforms are not considered synchronous since there may be a delayed receipt of these messages. Synchronous services are usually planned at a designated date/time. The exception is a crisis service, such as a telephone hotline, which provides a non-scheduled synchronous support. Crisis response is one of the benefits of a synchronous service. If a client expresses intent to harm themselves or others during a synchronous session, the counselor is live in the session with the client, and able to respond immediately using emergency guidelines previously established with the client.

Asynchronous platforms allow counseling to be conducted in delayed time, with the counselor and client responding to messages at any point in time. These platforms include email and text, as well as chat or instant messaging, and are also known as "store and forward" systems (Luxton et al., 2016). Video recordings that are stored and forwarded for client/counselor review are considered asynchronous services. Asynchronous services usually do not need to be scheduled in advance. It is recommended that informed consent documents define how often counselors will be checking and responding to messages, as well as expected time frames for client responses (Luxton et al., 2016). Asynchronous platforms are convenient for clients who are unable to designate a specific period in their day/week to receive counseling, but still benefit from communicating with a counselor. One of the risks of asynchronous services is responding to crisis situations. Clients may express harm to self or others in a message that is unseen for a period of time. This is mitigated through pre-established protocols for crisis (e.g., local emergency contacts, written expectations to contact emergency help line, call 911, etc.), in addition to establishing emergency contact guidelines with the client (Center for Credentialing in Education [CCE], 2016).

Blended platforms combine both synchronous and asynchronous services. TMH software systems combine modalities such as chat, email, and video conferencing. Like all platforms, blended platforms must be secure and maintain HIPAA compliance. Platforms such as Skype, FaceTime, and Google Handouts are generally not considered secure or HIPAA-compliant platforms, although new features continue to emerge. New software continues to be developed which allows counselors to conduct services in multiple modalities, while also including features such as billing, appointment scheduling, and notes. These software systems create a virtual, electronic "office," online, simulating services provided in a physical office space. It can be difficult for a counselor to decide which blended platform is right for their practice. Practitioners are urged to take advantage of trial versions, test systems fully with friends and colleagues, and compare systems to see which suits your needs. It is also recommended to obtain a Business Affiliation Agreement (BAA) with any technology vendor being utilized in your practice (Luxton et al., 2016).

Turnkey platforms remove much of the decision-making for distance counselors by providing a blended platform, network of providers, and pool of potential clients. Two of the largest turnkey distance counseling platforms in the United States (as of this publication) are BetterHelp™ and TalkSpace™. Counselors join the platform, participate in a screening process, and provide their license/credentials. Once hired as an independent contractor, counselors generally create their own informed consent document, counselor profile, and selected availability. Counselors select via which modality they will see clients, such as telephone, message, and/or video conferencing. They are then matched to clients they are licensed to serve based on skills, abilities, and client selection. Turnkey platforms offer various levels of support and training, and do not necessarily require the provider to have experience delivering distance services. It is not clear to what extent turnkey platforms screen clients for appropriateness to utilize

DC and TMH; however, emergency contact information is collected via these platforms and emergency protocols are established by most turnkey platforms.

MODALITIES

DC and TMH can be delivered via multiple modalities. The earliest documented TMH sessions utilized closed-circuit two-way televisions to provide psychiatric services in 1959 (Breen & Matusitz, 2010). Telephone counseling with non-professionals emerged from suicide hotlines in the 1950s (Hornblow, 1986). Today counselors deliver TMH and distance counseling via modalities such as telephone, email, text, chat, and videoconferencing. These modalities represent a sample of the most commonly used TMH delivery systems, but it is expected that DC and TMH modalities will continue to grow and evolve. It can be expected that some modalities will dissipate while others will emerge.

Telephone

One of the earliest modalities is telephone counseling. As stated, telephone crisis counseling emerged in the 1950s in London and was common in the United States by the 1970s (Hornblow, 1986). As counseling has evolved, telephones have evolved: from the wired and wall-mounted phones of the 1970s, to wireless phones of the 1980s, to cellular phones of the 1990s, to the mobile smartphones of the 2000s. In 2019, 96% of Americans owned a cellular phone. Eighty-one percent owned a smartphone, a significant increase from 35% of smartphone users in 2011 (Pew Research Group, 2019). Telephone counseling is now common, both for regular sessions and emergency consults. Depending on state licensing laws, telephone counseling may be used when a client cannot participate in their regular F2F session, or when the client needs immediate support outside of their normally scheduled session. It may also be used as the client's regular counseling modality (Reese et al., 2006). In earlier studies, telephone counseling was the preferred modality for TMH (Centore & Milacci, 2008; Reese et al., 2006).

Mobile phones can present security challenges. Not all mobile phones are secure and not all phones are able to be encrypted (Saunders & Osborn, 2016). Connectivity is also a challenge. When using hard-wire phones, speakers rarely had to worry about dropped calls. Signal strength of mobile telephone counseling, as well as encryption, is something that both counselors and clients will need to address if engaging in telephone counseling. Telephone counseling would be considered a synchronous service since it happens in real time for the client and counselor. Telephone counseling does not include telephone calls made for scheduling, changing, or canceling appointments, or for insurance information or logistical information.

Videoconferencing

Videoconferencing is quickly becoming one of the most widely utilized modality for TMH services (Lutxon et al., 2016), and is considered to be effective for various clinical issues (Cipoletta & Mocellin, 2018). Like telephone counseling, videoconferencing has had many evolutions. The earliest recorded TMH session utilized closed-circuit televisions, which closely resembled the videoconference sessions of today. Videoconference TMH services are delivered in multiple formats. In the **clinic-to-clinic** format, the session originates at one session, such as a major metropolitan hospital that houses many mental health specialists, and is transmitted to one or several satellite clinics. In this format, clients actually go to a community clinic to receive services from a provider located at the originating site. The benefit of clinic to clinic systems is that they tend to be more secure, and use both hardware and software dedicated to TMH delivery. Because the session is being delivered from one secure, confidential setting (e.g., hospital) to another (e.g., clinic) the counselor has more control over the session, and there are resources available at the clinic should a crisis arise (CCE, 2016). This is also sometimes referred to as the "hub and spoke" system, where the originating session is considered the hub (e.g., hospital) and the satellite locations are considered the spokes (e.g., clinics) (Luxton et al., 2016).

Another type of videoconferencing TMH is a direct-to-consumer model. In this model, a client receives TMH in a location of their choosing, as opposed to receiving services at a designated location, such as a clinic. Clients participate in TMH sessions from their home, office, or other secure and confidential location. In this model, the counselor is located in their formal office (such as a hospital, clinic, or agency) or in a home office of their private practice. Several software systems are available for purchase by either agencies or individuals to provide direct-to-consumer TMH counseling. There are concerns that clients may not use secure devices to receive these services, or that the setting they select may not be confidential. For example, people who participate in a TMH session on their work computer can potentially have their employer access anything on the computer (CCE, 2016). Similarly, participating in a counseling session at a local coffee shop using public Wi-Fi would not be considered a secure and confidential setting.

Counselors can also opt-in to turnkey platforms, a web-based software that provides videoconferencing, as well as other modalities, and join a network of providers as an independent contractor. These turnkey platforms usually have built-in encryption features and emergency contact methods. But like direct-to-consumer models, confidentiality and security are concerns. Videoconferencing services are primarily considered synchronous because they happen in live time, however some systems create video recordings. With these recordings, clients can participate in asynchronous communication where the client or counselor views a video on their own time. Additionally, live video sessions can be recorded for client and counselor to review at a later time, mimicking asynchronous services.

Email

Email counseling uses written word, as opposed to the spoken word of telephone and videoconferencing. Both the client and the counselor must be able to comfortably and appropriately communicate via typing, although newer software allows for talk-to-text features. The counselor and the client should both consider their computer skills before engaging in email counseling. The client and counselor must also consider their command of the preferred language used in session. Counselors and clients may be comfortable conducting a verbal session in a second language, but may be less comfortable communicating that language in writing. Some people prefer email counseling because it gives them time to process and review the other person's feedback before responding. This can be both a pro and a con of email counseling. Reflection allows the respondent to consider meaning and context before responding. But it also allows the respondent to self-edit, and may reduce the immediacy and genuineness of responses. Nonverbal communication may be lost via email counseling, yet some typed symbols can be used to portray emotion (e.g., CAPS = yelling or emphasizing words/feelings; use of emojis or emoticons; Recupero & Harms, 2016).

Email counseling creates an automatic transcript of the counseling session, which is also both a pro and con of email counseling (Recupero & Harms, 2016). The transcript can be helpful to both the counselor and client in remembering what was covered in each session. At the same time, email history creates an automatic transcript which is eligible to be surrendered in compliance with a court order. Most counselors, if called to testify or produce records in compliance with a court order, would not provide every detail of their counseling session (e.g., see American Counseling Association [ACA] code on minimal disclosures). Depending on the nature of the court order, a counselor may be required to submit an entire transcript, a redacted version, or simply their notes of the session. Some counselors may be uncomfortable with a verbatim recording of their sessions.

Like telephone counseling, email counseling is not to be confused with email exchanges regarding appointments and logistics. However, like telephone and videoconferencing, email counseling raises concerns with security and privacy. The most common, free email systems are not secure and/or encrypted. As a result, information sent via these email addresses has the potential of being hacked or read by third parties. People who engage in email counseling should be using a secure/encrypted email platform, password protections on their email and device, and ensuring that no other persons are reading their email. Using this example , emails sent on a work laptop or PC are able to be read/reviewed at the employer's discretion (Recupero & Harms, 2016). Code words are often created to ensure that the person sending the email is the person who is being serviced in counseling. Email counseling is typically considered an asynchronous service as the client and counselor need not be present at the same time to engage in counseling.

Text and Chat

Text and chat are growing modalities for counseling (Predmore et al., 2017). While considered asynchronous services, there is occasionally a sense of immediacy with texting that is not present in email communications. This urgency is reflected in the emergence of crisis text lines, where trained providers respond to texts from people in crisis that reach out via text, similar to crisis phone lines. Chat and instant messages are delivered through specific software, apps, or another platform, such as chat features on turnkey platforms or mobile applications. Similar to email communication, text and chat require written word, as opposed to spoken word. This provides the same pros and cons as email counseling, in that there is both time to reflect before responding and an automatic transcript of the session. Similar to email, nonverbal communication may be lost, yet the use of emojis and emoticons are helpful in portraying emotion via text and chat systems. Like email, both users must be comfortable communicating via text or chat, and must be proficient in doing so. Unlike email, responses may be more succinct due to the nature of communication via text/chat. In addition, text communication often includes abbreviations of words and key phrases, (e.g., omg = oh my god/gosh, ttyl = talk to you later). It is recommended that the counselor be familiar with this style of communication before engaging in text/chat sessions, and that the client understands these types of abbreviations before sending.

Security, like telephone, email, and videoconferencing, are also a concern with chat/text. Devices being used for text/chat must be secure and encrypted, and ideally not accessed by any other individual. Security features, such as code words and encryption should also be used with text/chat systems. Connectivity, like telephone and video conferencing may also be a concern. Low bandwidth may cause delayed messages, or may cause longer messages to be broken up into multiple texts and displayed out of order. Each of these possibilities need to be addressed with the client prior to engaging in text/chat counseling.

Emerging Technology

In the weeks following the COVID-19 shelter-in-place order, dozens of lesser-known (yet equally effective) technologies surfaced. While most of these technologies used the modalities already addressed, including videoconferencing, email, and chat, newer technologies are currently infusing additional modalities, such as gaming (Matthews & Coyle, 2016), virtual reality (Riva & Repetto, 2016; Tan, 2016), podcasting (Quiniones, 2016), blogging (Merz Nagel & Palumbo, 2016), or other resources, to provide DC and TMH services.

Exclusions

Counselors are encouraged to recognize what is not included as TMH and DC modalities. First, using social media to provide counseling services is not a modality to deliver DC and TMH. Social media can provide an avenue for counselors to market their services, share information about their practice, or publish their expertise. Some social media platforms provide referral mechanisms to help someone in crisis or provide a messaging feature. Some clients may even opt to share social media information with counselors during session. While some restrictions surrounding social media were lifted during the COVID-19 crisis, the delivery of counseling services via social media is discouraged, if not outright condemned. For example, Section A.5.e in the ACA code of ethics (A.5.e) states "Counselors are prohibited from engaging in personal virtual relationships with individuals with whom they have a current counseling relationship (e.g., through social media)" (ACA, 2014, p. 5). The ACA (H.6.a.) requires that practitioners keep separate personal and professional social media pages if they are using social media for professional purposes. These guidelines only scratch the surface of TMH and DC ethics, yet support the rationale for excluding social media as a modality to provide services.

Similarly, online blogs and email listserv are not included in TMH and DC modalities. It is the public nature of these forums, and the omission of direct, interchangeable communication between counselor and client, that exclude these forums as a DC modality. Blogs and listserv are often posted to public forums, or transmitted to individuals who opt-in based on interest. Even when listserv are housed within professional organizations, such as the American Counseling Association's *ACA Connect*, the nature of these conversations are public, often including a person's name, professional information, and photo. These forums provide exceptional resources for networking and information sharing, much like some social media platforms, but lack the direct communication, confidentiality, and privacy required for distance counseling. It should be noted that email listserv do not include individual or small group counseling emails directly between clients and counselor.

Websites, mobile apps, and self-help tools are not, in and of themselves, included as a modality of DC. Like social media, blogs, and listservs, these websites, apps, and self-help tools are available to the public based on interest, and lack direct communication between counselor and client. There are however certain websites, apps, and self-help tools that can provide information directly to a counselor on clients' coping and progress, such as apps for meditation and relaxation breathing. These tools may be used to supplement F2F or TMH counseling sessions, or may be used as standalone tools by a client. Be careful recommending mobile apps, websites, or self-help tools to your clients, particularly if you are unsure of the credentials of its creator, the security of the site/app/tool, and if the validity of the site/app/tool. The American Psychiatric Association publishes a mental health app rating system and evaluation tool on their website that helps clients and counselors determine if an app is reputable. [https://www.psychiatry.org/psychiatrists/practice/mental-health-apps]. While some professional organizations do include self-help sites and apps in their definitions of TMH, it is the lack of directed communication between a counselor and client that leads these modalities to be excluded from the discussion of TMH and DC in this book.

CERTIFICATIONS AND PROFESSIONAL ORGANIZATIONS

Professional organizations recognize the growth and value of DC and TMH practice. They acknowledge this growth by developing practice standards and ethical codes to guide practitioners' work. The Zur Institute compiles a listing of ethical and practice standards pertaining to TMH from 14 leading organizations, including the American Association of Marriage and Family Therapists, American Counseling Association, American Medical Association, American Mental Health Counselors Association, American

Psychiatric Association, American Psychological Association, American Telemedicine Association, Association of Canadian Psychology Regulatory Organizations, Association of Social Work Boards, California Association of Marriage and Family Therapists, California Board of Behavioral Sciences, Canadian Psychological Association, National Association of Social Workers, and National Board of Certified Counselors (Zur, 2019). While this list is extensive, it excludes non-mental health organizations who have also adapted their codes and practices to address technology, including the National Career Development Association (NCDA), American School Counselors Association (ASCA), and NAADAC (formerly the National Association of Alcohol and Drug Addiction Counselors).

Ethical guidance from these organizations supports the broad utility and acceptance for distance services, but fails to provide practitioners with training to practice TMH. Counseling practitioners have expressed desire for training in distance modalities (Baird et al., 2018; Centore & Milacci, 2008; Cipoletta & Mocellin, 2018; Perle et al., 2012; Simms et al., 2011). While training and certificate programs exist, few have been endorsed by professional organizations and there remains concern and criticism that these training programs lack universal content (Anthony, 2015; Colbow, 2013).

The CCE, an affiliate of the National Board of Certified Counselors (NBCC), launched the DCC credential in 2003 (Malone, 2007). The DCC credential required (a) a master's degree in counseling or a counseling related field, (b) a license to practice professional counseling (or a certificate as a Nationally Certified Counselor), (c) adherence to the NBCC Standards Regarding the Provision of Distance Professional Services, and (d) completion of an approved DCC training program (CCE, 2014). The credential also required an application fee, renewal fee, and ongoing professional development. In 2018, DCC holders were notified by the CCE that the DCC credential would be eliminated. DCC holders were given the option to transition to a new credential, the Board Certified Telemental Health Provider (BC-TMH), by completing additional training and applying for the credential.

The BC-TMH is now the distance credential promoted by CCE. To become a BC-TMH provider, candidates must have (a) a license in a behavioral health field or a certificate from a wide range of counseling and related professions, such as substance abuse, pastoral counseling, rehabilitation, school counseling, and many others outlined at www.cce-global.org/Assets/BCTMH/QualifyingCertificationsandCredentials.pdf. Individuals must also (b) complete the Telemental Health Professional Training Series. This training is available for purchase through the CCE. Finally, (c) applicants must disclose any legal, criminal or professional charges. The credential also requires an application fee, renewal fee, and ongoing professional development.

The transition to the BC-TMH expanded the type of practitioner that can earn the credential beyond professional counselors. While NBCC has not officially endorsed the BC-TMH for DC and TMH, its affiliation with the CCE suggests their approval of the credential and its training content. The BC-TMH requirements page links directly to the Telemental Health Professional Training Series through the CCE website, yet the required training page provides other approved training programs. Although other certificate and training programs exist, professional organizations have not formally endorsed specific training programs for DC and TMH. The hesitancy of professional organizations to endorse specific programs may be due to lack of uniformity and consistency. Appendix 2.A outlines four different TMH training certificates from four different organizations. These training programs range from 9 to 36 hours of training, and cost anywhere from $150 to nearly $1,500. While the content of each training program is valuable, the counselor is left to determine how much training they wish to purchase and which training is most relevant to their practice.

Some states have specific requirements in order to practice TMH. The law firm Epstein Becker Green publishes a guide of telemental health practice laws across 50 states and Washington, DC. The 2017 guide is available as a PDF on their website and the 2019 guide is available as a mobile application downloadable for iPhone, iPad, and android. The guide outlines telemental health laws for psychiatrists, psychologists, social workers, counselors, marriage and family therapists, and advanced practice registered nurses in all 50 states and Washington, DC. For each specialization (e.g., counselor, social worker), the guide provides the state authority, the scope of practice, the licensing requirements, the practitioner–patient relationship, prescribing authority, and accepted modalities, quoting the state legislation directing such activities. The guide also includes key terms and guidance on privacy/confidentiality, minors, follow-up care, coverage and reimbursement, and controlled substances (Epstein Becker Green Law, 2019). In addition to guides such as these, counselors and practitioners are encouraged to check with their state licensing and regulatory boards to ensure that they are meeting the certification and training requirements prior to engaging in practice.

COUNCIL ON THE ACCREDITATION OF COUNSELING AND RELATED EDUCATION PROGRAMS STANDARDS AND TECHNOLOGY

The Council on the Accreditation of Counseling and Related Education Programs (CACREP) is arguably the largest accrediting body of counselor education programs, with over 850 masters and doctoral program accreditations approved or in process (CACREP Directory, 2019). These programs are graduating thousands of professional counselors into the field of school counseling, clinical mental health counseling, career counseling, clinical rehabilitation counseling, and other counseling specializations. The 2016 CACREP standards are the most recent standards published, with the prior standards being published in 2009. The 2016 standards are now being utilized in all accreditation decisions. The standards aim to "promote a unified counseling profession" (p. 3). Thus it is logical to turn to the CACREP standards for guidance on educating and training the counseling workforce in DC.

Technology is addressed both explicitly and implicitly throughout the CACREP standards, however the terms "distance counseling," "telemental health," "TMH, or other TMH terms are not explicitly stated in the 2016 standards. Explicitly, the term "technology" is mentioned in section 2) Professional Practice. Under section 2.F.1., Professional Counseling Orientation and Ethical Practice, standard 2.F.1.j. requires programs to address "technology's impact on the counseling profession" (CACREP, 2016, p. 11). Similarly, in Section 2.F.5. Counseling and Helping Relationships, standard 2.F.5.e. requires programs to address "the impact of technology on the counseling process" (CACREP, 2016, p. 12). Thus counselor education programs are required to address the *impact* of technology on the counseling process, but not how to use technology in the counseling process. Standard 2.F.5.f. requires programs to address "ethically and culturally relevant strategies for establishing and maintaining in-person and *technology-assisted relationships*" which asserts that technology-assisted relationships exist and require attention. The only other mention of technology is Section 2.F.4. Career Development, where standard 2.F.4.c. requires programs to address "process for identifying and using career, a vocational, educational, occupational and labor market information resources, technology, and information systems" (p. 12).

Implicitly, technology is addressed in section 5) Entry-Level Specialty Areas, although not aimed at TMH or DC. Section 5.D.2q. Clinical Rehabilitation Counseling requires instruction on "assistive technology to reduce or eliminate barriers and functional limitations," as well as 5.D.3.a. addressing "assessments for assistive technology needs" (p. 27). Within these contexts, assistive technology refers to a clinical intervention to assist a person with a disability, as opposed to a counseling modality of practice. Despite the direct omissions of TMH and DC language, there are references in the CACREP standards that suggest inclusion. For example, section 2.B. Professional Counseling Identity Foundation reads "program objectives (1) reflect current knowledge and projected needs concerning counseling practice in a multicultural and pluralistic society" and 2.B. Professional Counseling Curriculum reads "current counseling related research is infused in the curriculum" (p. 10). As DC and TMH continue to grow in relation to practice and research, counselor education programs will need to critically examine the content of their programs to ensure that they are graduating ethically competent counselors who are trained in technology's impact on the profession. These changes are particularly relevant post-COVID-19, in which graduate students in counselor education programs were suddenly faced with practicing via distance modalities.

DC and TMH training continue to lack unified standards. The 2016 CACREP standards are unlikely to provide the depth of content required to effectively engage in TMH practice. However, the next revision of CACREP standards is scheduled to be released in 2023, which may address DC and TMH in more detail. For those seeking clarification and guidance, counselors are required to seek external resources, such as this book or formal certificate programs, in order to broaden their understanding of ethical and effective distance counseling practices.

CONCLUSION

DC and TMH include a multitude of terms and concepts not often utilized in F2F counseling. This book uses both DC and TMH, since some counseling specialties may not work with mental health concerns. Critical concepts for DC/TMH practitioners include HIPAA guidelines and utilizing encrypted devices. DC/TMH takes place in both planned and unplanned settings, as well as on multiple platforms, including synchronous, asynchronous, blended, and turnkey platforms. Multiple modalities may be utilized for DC/TMH interventions including telephone, email, videoconferencing, text and chat; other technologies continue to emerge daily. While not specifically utilized for DC/TMH interventions, other technologies such as social media, mobile apps, online blogs, email listserves, and self-help websites may also support and impact counseling interactions. While there are no unified training standards, there are a variety of training programs available. While the most recent CACREP (2016) standards do not require training in DC/TMH, counselors must be aware of state laws that impact DC/TMH interventions in their state, and the state where their clients/students are located.

REFERENCES

American Counseling Association. (2014). *2014 ACA code of ethics*. https://www .counseling.org/resources/aca-code-of-ethics.pdf

Anthony, K. (2015). Training therapists to work effectively online and offline within digital culture. *British Journal of Guidance & Counselling, 43*, 36–42. https://doi .org/10.1080/03069885.2014.924617

Baird, M. B., Whitney, L., & Caedo, C. E. (2018). Experiences and attitudes among psychiatric mental health advanced practice nurses in the use of telemental health: Results of an online survey. *Journal of the American Psychiatric Nurses Association, 24*(3), 235–240. https://doi.org/10.1177/1078390317717330

Breen, G. M., & Matusitz, J. (2010). An evolutionary examination of telemedicine: A health and computer-mediated communication perspective. *Social Work Public Health, 25*(1), 59–71. https://doi.org/10.1080/19371910902911206

Center for Credentialing in Education. (2014). *Distance credentialed counselor application package.* https://www.cce-global.org/Assets/DCC/DCCapp.pdf

Center for Credentialing in Education. (2016). Differences between a clinic-to-clinic video meeting and a home-home based TMH video meeting. *Telemental Health Professional Training Series, Module 5: Best practices in video telemental health.* Author.

Centore, A. J., & Milacci, A. (2008). A study of mental health counselor's use and perspectives on distance counseling. *Journal of Mental Health Counseling, 30,* 267–282. https://doi.org/10.17744/mehc.30.3.q871r684n863u75r

Cipoletta, S., & Mocellin, D. (2018). Online counseling: An exploratory survey of Italian psychologists' attitudes toward new ways of interaction. *Psychotherapy Research, 28,* 909–924. https://doi.org/10.1080/10503307.2016.1259533

Colbow, A. J. (2013). Looking to the future: Integrating telemental health therapy in to psychologist training. *Training and Education in Professional Psychology, 7*(3), 155–165. https://doi.org/10.1037/a0033454

Council on the Accreditation of Counseling and Related Education Programs. (2016). *2016 CACREP Standards and Glossary.* http://www.cacrep.org/wp-content/uploads/2018/05/2016-Standards-with-Glossary-5.3.2018.pdf

Council on the Accreditation of Counseling and Related Education Programs. (2019). *Directory.* https://www.cacrep.org/directory

Dryman, M. T., McTeague, L. M., Olino, T. M., & Heimberg, R. G. (2017). Evaluation of an open-access CBT-based internet program for social anxiety: Patterns of use, retention, and outcomes. *Journal of Consulting & Clinical Psychology, 85,* 988–1000. https://doi.org/10.1037/ccp0000232

Epstein Becker Green Law. (2019). *Telemental Health Laws [mobile application software].* https://play.google.com/store

Epstein Becker Green Law. (2020). *Telemental health laws update.* https://www.ebglaw.com/covid-19-telemental-health-laws-update/

Hornblow, A. R. (1986). The evolution and effectiveness of telephone counseling services. *Hospital and Community Psychiatry, 37,* 731–733. https://doi.org/10.1176/ps.37.7.731

Luxton, D. D., Nelson, E., & Maheu, M. M. (2016). A practitioner's guide to telemental health: *How to conduct legal, ethical, and evidence-based telepractice.* American Psychological Association.

Malone, J. F. (2007). Understanding distance counseling. In J. E. Malone, R. M., Miller, & G. R. Walz (Eds.), *Distance counseling: Expanding the counselor's reach and impact.* Counseling Outfitters.

Matthews, M., & Coyle D. (2016). The role of gaming in mental health. In S. Goss., K. Anthony., L. Sykes Stretch, & D. Merz Nagel (Eds.), *Technology in mental health: Applications in practice, supervision, and training* (2nd ed). Charles C. Thomas Publishing.

Mehrotra, A., Huskamp, H. A., Souza, J., Uscher-Pines, L., Rose, S., Landon, B. E., Jena, A. B., & Busch, A. B. (2017). Rapid growth in mental health telemedicine use among rural Medicare beneficiaries, wide variation across states. *Health Affairs, 36,* 909–917. https://doi.org/10.1377/hlthaff.2016.1461

Merz Nagel, D., & Palumbo, G. (2016). The role of blogging in mental health. In S. Goss., K. Anthony., L. Sykes Stretch, & D. Merz Nagel (Eds.), *Technology in mental health: Applications in practice, supervision, and training* (2nd ed.). Charles C. Thomas Publishing.

Myers, K., & Turvey, C. L. (Eds.). (2013). *Telemental health: Clinical and administrative foundations for evidence-based practice.* Elsevier.

Perle, J. G., Langsam, L. C., Randel, A., Lutchman, S., Levine, A B., Odland, A. P., Nierenberg, B., & Marker, C. D. (2012). Attitudes toward psychological telehealth: Current and future clinical psychologists opinions of internet-based interventions. *Journal of Clinical Psychology, 69,* 100–113. https://doi.org/10.1002/jclp.21912

Pew Research Group. (12 June, 2019). *Internet and technology; Mobile fact sheet.* https://www.pewinternet.org/fact-sheet/mobile

Predmore, Z., Ramchand, R., Ayer, L., Kotzias, V., Engel, C., Ebener, P., Kemp, J. E., Karras, E., & Haas, G. L. (2017). Expanding suicide crisis services to text and chat. *Crisis, 38*(4), 255–260. https://doi.org/10.1027/0227-5910/a000460

Pruitt, L. D., Luxton, D. D., & Shore, P. (2014). Additional clinical benefits of home-based telemental health treatments. *Professional Psychology: Research and Practice, 45,* 340–346. https://doi.org/10.1037/a0035461

Quinones, M. A. (2016). The use of podcasting in mental health. In S. Goss., K. Anthony., L. Sykes Stretch, & D. Merz Nagel (Eds.), *Technology in mental health: Applications in practice, supervision, and training* (2nd ed). Charles C. Thomas Publishing.

Recupero, P. R., & Harms, S. (2016). Using email to conduct a therapeutic relationship. In S. Goss., K. Anthony., L. Sykes Stretch, & D. Merz Nagel (Eds.), *Technology in mental health: Applications in practice, supervision, and training* (2nd ed.). Charles C. Thomas Publishing.

Reese, R. J., Conoley, C. W., & Brossert, D. F. (2006). The attractiveness of telephone counseling: An empirical investigation of client perceptions. *Journal of Counseling & Development, 84,* 54–60. https://doi.org/10.1002/j.1556-6678.2006.tb00379.x

Riva, G., & Repetto, C. (2016). Using virtual reality immersion therapeutically. In S. Goss., K. Anthony., L. Sykes Stretch, & D. Merz Nagel (Eds.), *Technology in mental health: Applications in practice, supervision, and training* (2nd ed.). Charles C. Thomas Publishing.

Saunders, D. E., & Osborn, D. S. (2016). Using the telephone for conducting a therapeutic relationship. In S. Goss., K. Anthony., L. Sykes Stretch, & D. Merz Nagel (Eds.), *Technology in mental health: Applications in practice, supervision, and training* (2nd ed.). Charles C. Thomas Publishing.

Simms, D. C., Gibson, K., & O'Donnell, S. (2011). To use or not to use: Clinicians' perceptions of telemental health. *Canadian Psychology, 52*, 41–51. https://doi.org/10.1037/a0022275

Tan, L. (2016). The use of virtual reality for peer support. In S. Goss., K. Anthony., L. Sykes Stretch, & D. Merz Nagel (Eds.), *Technology in mental health: Applications in practice, supervision, and training* (2nd ed.). Charles C. Thomas Publishing.

U.S. Department of Commerce's National Institutes for Standards of Technology. (n.d.). *Computer security resource center: Glossary (encryption).* https://csrc.nist.gov/glossary/term/encryption

U.S. Department of Health and Human Services. (1996). *Health Insurance Portability and Accountability Act.* https://aspe.hhs.gov/report/health-insurance-portability-and-accountability-act-1996

U.S. Department of Health and Human Services. (2017). *HIPAA for professionals.* https://www.hhs.gov/hipaa/for-professionals/index.html

Zur, O. (2019). *Professional association codes of ethics and guidelines on telemental health, e-therapy, digital ethics, and social media.* https://www.zurinstitute.com/ethics-of-telehealth/#top

Appendix 2.A

TABLE 2.A COMPARISON OF TELEMENTAL HEALTH CERTIFICATES (AUGUST 2019)

CERTIFICATE TITLE; HOURS; COST; WEBSITE	SELECTED CONTENT
Board Certified TMH Provider (BC-TMH); 9 hrs; $382.50; https://www.cce-global.org/ credentialing/bctmh/training	• Introduction to TMH • Presentation Skills for TMH • HIPAA Compliance for TMH • Best Practices in Video TMH • Crisis Planning and Protocols in Video TMH • Choosing and Using Technology in TMH • Orienting Clients/Patients to TMH • Direct-to-Consumer TMH • TMH Settings and Care Coordination
TMH Training Certificate; 10.5; $350; https://www. telementalhealthtraining.com	• Introduction to TMH • Legal Aspects of TMH • Ethics of Using Technology in Behavioral Health • HIPAA Compliance for Mental Health Professionals • Ethical, Legal, and Clinical Aspects of Selecting Technology • Emergency Management Planning for TMH • Screening for Fit for TMH Services • Ethical and Clinical Skills of Video and Phone Sessions
Telebehavioral Health Institute (3 levels: Basic, Level I and Level II certification); **Basic** (6 hrs; $149); **Level I** (15 hrs; $370); **Level II** (36 hrs; $1,495); https://telehealth.org/ telebehavioral-health-certificate	**Basic** 1. Essential Concepts 2. Evidence-Based Models 3. Technology 4. Laws and Ethics **Level I (Plus Basic)** 1. Legal/Ethical Issues I: Rules, Regulations and Risk Management 2. Telephone and Videoconferencing in Telepractice 3. Advanced Clinical Telepractice Issues (Handling Online Emergencies) **Level II (Plus Basic and Level I)** 1. Legal/Ethical Issues II: Best Practices and Informed Consent 2. 6 Fundamentals for Setting Up Your Video-Based Office

(continued)

TABLE 2.A COMPARISON OF TELEMENTAL HEALTH CERTIFICATES (AUGUST 2019) (*CONTINUED*)

CERTIFICATE TITLE; HOURS; COST; WEBSITE	SELECTED CONTENT
	3. Telehealth Documentation and Administrative Compliance: Legal, Ethical and Other Requirements 4. Texting and Behavioral Health Course Basic Dos and Don'ts 5. Telehealth Reimbursement Strategies: Increasing Authorization and Payment
Zur Institute Certificate in TMH and Digital Ethics; 26 hrs; $156; https://www.zurinstitute.com/course/certificate-in-telemental-health	• Historical and Contemporary Context of TMH Standards Development • Relevant Laws, Regulations and Ethics Codes • Assess One's Own Competencies for Conducting TMH • Present on Video in a Clinically and Technologically Effective Manner • HIPAA • Safely Managing TMH Client Crises and Technology Failures • Choose Email and Texting Technology That Is Appropriate for Professional Practice • Utilize the Unique Advantages, Such as Leveraging Online Disinhibition Effect and Asynchronous Interventions, for Clinical Effectiveness • Basic Issues in Performing Couples, Family, and Group Therapy by TMH • Choose Appropriate Tools for Practice • Establish and Maintain a TMH Practice That Is Legal, Ethical, and Effective • Specific Skills to Use with Telepsychology • Barriers of Using Telepsychology With Psychoanalysis • Telepsychology Principles to Experiential, Emotional and Creative Psychotherapy • Telepsychology for Clients With Financial-Related Disorders • Using Smartphone Technology With Alcoholic Clients • Using Telepsychology to Treat PTSD • Social Media and Several Popular Social Media Sites and Services • Distinguish Between One's Personal and Professional Activities on the Internet • Ethical Challenges That May Arise From Engaging in Activities on the Internet • Strategies for Minimizing Risk of Ethical violations on the Internet • Use of Email, Record-Keeping, and Mobile Computing Devices to Prevent Confidentiality Breaches

(*continued*)

TABLE 2.A COMPARISON OF TELEMENTAL HEALTH CERTIFICATES (AUGUST 2019) *(CONTINUED)*

CERTIFICATE TITLE; HOURS; COST; WEBSITE	SELECTED CONTENT
	• Social Media Policy for One's Office to Address Potential boundary Issues With Clients • Different Approaches and Attitudes Towards Social Networking Between Therapists and Clients • Discuss the Relevant Ethical Issues as They Pertain to Therapists' Websites and Social Networking Profiles

3

Ethics and Professionalism in Telemental Health

INTRODUCTION

Counselors are exposed to ethics early in their professional training. Professional ethics and orientation to counseling are usually among the earliest courses offered to counselors-in-training, if not the first courses in a counselor training program. Similarly, from the moment most counselors-in-training begin their program, they are required to join a professional organization, such as the American Counseling Association (ACA), the American School Counselors Association (ASCA), the American Mental Health Counseling Association (AMHCA), or others. This student membership helps to solidify identity in the counseling profession, while often including liability insurance required in most counselor training programs.

An early focus on ethics, professionalism, and liability is appropriate for several reasons. Before beginning any practice, counselors-in-training must be aware of the ethical guidelines for professional practice in order to avoid harm to themselves and to clients. Similarly, early exposure allows counselors-in-training to reflect on these ethics, and determine if becoming a counselor is appropriate for their needs, interests, and aspirations. It's not uncommon for a student to determine that counseling is not a "fit" for them after learning about the profession and its expectations. Finally, early exposure to law and ethics allows counselors-in-training to be aware of risk and liability inherent in the practice of counseling.

Distance counseling (DC) and telemental health (TMH) also require exposure to ethics and professionalism prior to practice. Before exploring the "how to" of TMH or diving into DC strategies, it's critical to understand the ethics and professionalism of TMH for the same reasons mentioned previously: avoiding harm, determining appropriateness, and awareness of risk and/or liability. During the COVID-19 pandemic, the rapid shift to TMH practice may not have allowed counselors to fully explore their ethical obligations when practicing in distance modalities. This chapter focuses on elements of ethical codes that address DC and TMH. The TMH counselor, however, must adhere to all elements of these ethical codes, not strictly those discussed in the chapter.

COUNSELING ETHICAL CODES

The National Board of Certified Counselors (NBCC) published the *Standards for Ethical Practice of WebCounseling* in 1997, which is often considered one of the earliest published guides on conducting TMH and DC. These guidelines "give the novice online counselor a vision of some of the professional, ethical, and legal pitfalls that might exist" and "give counselors and other behavioral health professionals the direction needed to minimize risk and danger to WebCounselor and WebClient alike" (Bloom, 1997, p. 2). Since then, a multitude of professional counseling organizations have published ethical guidelines pertaining to DC, TMH, technology, and Internet-based services. More recently, NBCC published the *Policy Regarding Provision of Distance Professional Services* (NBCC, 2016), which is specifically written for Nationally Certified Counselors (NCC). This document mirrors the ACA Code of Ethics, yet also contains unique content specific to distance practice.

The ACA serves as the world's primary professional development organization for profession counselors of all practices (ACA, n.d.). The *2014 ACA Code of Ethics* includes an entire section, added since the 2005 code, dedicated to DC and TMH. Specifically, Section H. Distance Counseling, Technology, and Social Media, outlines standards for the professional counselor. Even for counselors not practicing via distance modalities, the introduction to Section H indicates that all professional counselors recognize DC as a modality, understand technology's impact on the profession, and be aware of DC resources available to the public. Regardless of one's personal opinion or practice of TMH, all counselors are expected to understand potential concerns of distance counseling, social media, and technology in an effort to protect clients (ACA, 2014). Throughout this chapter, specific sections of the ACA code will be indicated in parentheses.

Counselor Competence

First and foremost, counselors are instructed to (H1a) be competent in their use of technology in their practice, specifically in relation to their technical skills, legal, and ethical issues (ACA, 2014). Counselors who wish to engage in TMH practice must first have the technical skills to utilize technology in this manner, and second, have the clinical skills to engage in counseling in a distance setting. Many counselors mistakenly assume that because they have technical skills and they also have counseling skills, they automatically possess the skills to conduct counseling via technology. In fact, multiple studies demonstrate that practitioners possess a sense of confidence in their ability to conduct distance sessions despite having limited training and practice in DC (Baird et al., 2018; Cipoletta & Mocellin, 2018). Practicing DC and TMH requires training and competence, both on how to conduct TMH sessions, as well as how to use TMH technology. This book addresses how to conduct TMH sessions, yet based on the varying and changing nature of technology, this chapter will only address technological concepts, as opposed to specific software systems.

Telemental Health Laws

Counselors engaging in DC and TMH must (H1b) be aware of all laws and statutes pertaining to the use of TMH. One way in which practitioners can learn their state's specific guidelines is to confer with the licensing and certification boards, specifically entities issuing mental health counseling licenses and/or school counseling certificates. If a professional counselor is operating as a practitioner not governed by a state licensing board, such as a career counselor or a rehabilitation counselor, it is recommended that the practitioner confer with the professional and national organizations that oversee their credentials in order to learn of any laws, statutes, recommendations, or guidelines pertaining to distance practice. The law firm Epstein Becker Green (2020) publishes the *50-State Survey of Telemental/Telebehavioral Health,* as well as a mobile app (2019), which is updated regularly with laws pertaining to TMH for a variety of mental health professionals, including professional counselors, social workers, psychologists, and others. While these resources are incredibly valuable, the most recent information should be obtained from state licensing and certification boards. NBCC Standard 3 also requires that counselors be aware of and adhere to legal regulations (NBCC, 2016).

Informed Consent

The informed consent document is one of the most critical elements to the delivery of TMH and DC. Like all informed consent documents, the TMH informed consent document must be presented in a manner that the client can understand, be presented in written and verbal formats with opportunities for questions, and be revisited throughout the treatment (ACA, 2014). Like all informed consents, the TMH informed consent should include items such as the purpose of counseling, limitations of confidentiality, pros and cons of engaging in counseling, counselor qualifications, and referral needs (ACA, 2014). It may also include information on fees, confidentiality, records, and potential changes in treatment. However, the addition of technology into the counseling relationship warrants specific attention. The ACA code specifies that the TMH informed consent document include elements such as counselors training in DC, physical location and contact information, as well as the risks of receiving counseling via DC/TMH. The informed consent should also address how the counselor will respond to technology failures, how soon they will respond to messages, and any emergency protocols for when the client cannot reach the counselor. Other important elements may include time zones, language/culture differences, insurance and payment issues, as well as social media (ACA, 2014, pp. 17–18). Similarly, NBCC counselors provide clients with a written document outlining considerations for distance practice, including items such as the modality and technological needs for DC, as well as if the modality is appropriate for the client's goal (NBCC, 2016). NBCC also requires that the document include concerns pertaining to confidentiality, privacy, technological failure, response time, and other relevant information that will assist the client in determining if they wish to engage in DC (NBCC, 2016).

The physical distance between the counselor and the client creates a new standard of practice. In face-to-face (F2F) settings, counselors need not specify anticipated response times, time zone differences, or protocols for technology failures. The distance counselor must prepare client alternatives for technology failure. Examples of such failures include how and when the counselor would contact the client if technology were to fail mid-session, if one party was unable to connect, or if the connection is abruptly terminated. These issues must be outlined in the informed consent before the client actually engages in distance practice. Other areas, such as emergency procedures, security and encryption, and confidentiality, are also included.

Client Verification

Anyone who has ever used a shared or public computer and realized that someone failed to sign out of their personal email account can understand the importance of client verification. In those circumstances, someone (who is not the owner of the email account) could send emails impersonating the true email address holder, causing potential damage for the email holder or their contacts. Similarly, anyone who has ever had to locate someone in a public place with only their name and no other information can understand the uncertainty of wondering if they've found the correct person. Virtual counseling relationships create the same risk and uncertainty. It is for that reason that counselors are required (H.3.) to verify client identity both in the beginning of counseling and throughout the process. Since requests for DC will come via email or telephone, the counselor may have never met the client in a F2F setting. NBCC's Standard 15 also requires client verification. It may be appropriate for the first counseling session be in person, whenever possible, yet based on geographic distance, meeting F2F is not always an option.

Client verification is conducted in a variety of ways. For example, a counselor has never met their client, John Doe, before. The client signs on to the video conference session saying "Hello, I'm John Doe." Does the counselor really know that the person on the screen is John Doe? Client verification is conducted by asking the client to send a copy of a government issued photo ID, which the counselor verifies and matches to the name and face of the person speaking.

Counselors can check the address to ensure it matches information from insurance providers or other sources. Counselors can also ask the client to verify pieces of information such as address or date of birth. Email and phone sessions also require verification. It is recommended that clients and counselors create a system, such as use of a code word, numbers, or image that is presented at the beginning of each session (ACA, 2014). Clients and counselors then start each verbal or typed session with that code word/corresponding response in an effort to confirm the identity of the client they are speaking with. While none of these systems are impervious to foul play or mal-intent, they demonstrate that the counselor has engaged in ethical best practices and made efforts to verify identity. These procedures should be used regularly and documented throughout their treatment.

Distance Counseling Relationship

If anyone has ever misinterpreted the meaning behind someone's text or email, or perhaps had one's own communication misconstrued, then they understand how these miscommunications can be exacerbated in a DC relationship. ACA requires that counselors explain these communication differences (H.4.f) to clients considering engaging in DC.

Counselors must ensure that distance modalities are the right fit for the clients they serve, which is also stipulated by NBCC's Standard 7. In order to determine if the client is appropriate for DC, the counselor must assess the person's cognitive, emotional, physical, intellectual, and technological functioning to engage in DC (H.4.e), as well as if the person has access to technology (H.4.e). Counselors help clients understand the benefits and limits of distance relationships (H.4.a) as well as potential boundary issues (H.4.b.). When DC is not appropriate, the counselor provides or seeks to provide assistance in identifying appropriate F2F services (H.4.c.).

Records

Clients who engage in DC must ensure that their records are secure and that the client's confidentiality is protected through encryption and storage of records (H.5.a). Counselors would need to follow appropriate Health Insurance Portability and Accountability Act of 1996 (HIPAA), electronic protected health information (ePHI), and Family Educational Rights and Privacy Act (FERPA) guidelines depending on their work setting. For counselors who maintain websites, these sites must maintain links to professional licensure boards to verify credentials (H.5.b), ensure that all electronic links are working (H.5.c), and ensure that websites are appropriate for multicultural and disability considerations (H.5.d). The Americans with Disabilities Act (ADA) website, managed by the United States Department of Justice, Civil Rights Division, publishes guidelines for website ADA compliance (2003). NBCC also requires that counselors create a backup system for communications and records that is encrypted (Standard 6), as well as engage in practices to protect client information from unauthorized access (Standard 9) (NBCC, 2016).

Social Media

ACA requires that, if counselors elect to utilize social media for their professional practice, they create separate personal and professional profiles (H.6.a) before doing so. Social media policies must be clearly outlined in informed consent documents (H.6.b). Social medial policies may vary based on specialization. For example, a mental health counselor's social media policy may state that they will not connect with clients/students on any social media platforms. A school counselor's policy might state that they will not connect with any student or parent on social media platforms. A career counselor's policy might allow connections on LinkedIn, but no other social media platforms. These are only examples, yet most social media policies should state that counselors will respect the privacy of their students'/clients' social media content (H.6.c). This means that counselors are not engaging in searches of clients on social media, or viewing client's social media content without permission. An exception would be if a client wants to show something to a counselor and voluntarily presents social media content to the counselor during session. The ACA (H.6.d.) and NBCC (Standard 13) both require that counselors not share confidential information via social media.

It is important to note that ACA (A.5.e.) specifically prohibits clients from having a personal virtual relationship with the clients they serve. Virtual relationship is defined as "engaging in a relationship via technology or social media that blurs the professional boundary" (Kaplan et al., 2015, p. 114). These boundary issues should be outlined and discussed with your clients prior to treatment, as well as the prohibition of virtual relationships. It is required that they be included in informed consent documents, such that clients recognize the policy is universal, and not personal. As Michelle Wade stated when the ACA 2014 codes were released, "This would include friending. . . ., it is a boundary issue. You wouldn't be friends with your clients face-to-face, so you should not be friends with your clients in a virtual setting either" (Kaplan et al., 2015).

This cursory review of the ACA and NBCC codes of ethics begins to demonstrate the depth of ethical issues present in TMH and DC practice. Counselors are encouraged to fully review the ACA codes, NBCC standards, and any ethical guidelines for counseling specializations they practice. Additionally, other helping professions such as social workers, psychologists, and psychiatrists have also published guidelines pertaining to TMH and DC. The Zur Institute (2019) maintains a comprehensive website with links to the ethical codes of most professional organizations pertaining to TMH, DC, and social media.

LICENSURE AND CREDENTIALING

One appealing aspect of DC and TMH is the ability to access clients and students in any location, including rural populations (Imig, 2014) and those who struggle to attend F2F counseling (Dryman et al., 2017). However, the ability to access a client or student does not equate to the ability to treat that individual. While states have clear geographic boundaries, the Internet is quite literally boundless. Licensure laws dictate that counselors may only practice within their professional competence. Yet TMH creates the possibility for unlicensed professionals to gain access to individuals that they are unqualified to serve.

Licensed Counselors

Professional counseling licensure is typically managed by state organizations. Professional counseling licensure now includes all 50 states in the United States, as well as the District of Columbia, Puerto Rico, and Guam, and is managed by 53 separate entities (ACA, 2020). Despite efforts to create a uniform standard for the counseling profession (Gerig, 2018), licensure standards vary from state to state. What is considered acceptable education, experience, or examination in one state, may be insufficient in another. Despite these differences, Licensed Professional Counselors (LPC), also known as Licensed Mental Health Counselors (LMHCs) and other terms, have the ability to fill the gap in health professional shortage areas (HPSA) that lack mental health services, including California, Texas, Michigan, and Arizona (Health Resources and Services Administration [HRSA], 2019). These large states, such as Alaska, California, and Texas, as well as rural areas such as the Dakotas, Wyoming, and Montana, benefit from accessing licensed counselors anywhere in the state. It is often presumed that counselors are unable to practice across state lines without a license in that state, although state regulations may vary. For example, North Carolina dictates that a counselor licensed in North Carolina who provides services out of state, must be sure they are complying with licensing laws in that state (Epstein Becker Green, 2019). Several other states follow this model. Thus the onus is on the counselor to conduct a thorough review of licensing laws where their clients are located.

Additional Requirements

A license alone, however, may not be sufficient for TMH practice in all states. Few states specify the need for additional credentials in order to practice TMH, yet other requirements still exist. Alaska, for example, requires that practitioners engaging in TMH register their business as a telemedicine business. West Virginia requires that counselors practicing TMH adhere to the ACA Code of Ethics and the NBCC Provisions for Distance Professional Services. Some states may use different language or definitions. Montana, for example, includes telephonic and video conferencing in their definition of direct client contact (Epstein Becker Green, 2019), while other states may not. Among these inconsistencies, the underlying message is that counselors must know and adhere to the licensing requirements in their own state, as well as those of any states in which their clients are located. A final concern for LPCs engaging in TMH is insurance reimbursement, as not all insurance providers recognize DC as a reimbursable practice, or will vary based on the location of the counselor and client (American Telemedicine Association [ATA], 2013). In the wake of COVID-19, many insurance companies lifted restrictions for TMH services (America's Health Insurance Plans [AHIP], 2020), yet it remains to be seen how long these approvals will last for mental health providers.

Nonlicensed Counselors

Not all professional counselors require a license. Certain counseling professions such as career counseling or rehabilitation counseling are not managed by state licensing boards. Career counselors may elect to earn an optional credential such as Global Career Development Facilitator (GCDF) or a Certified Career Counselor (CCC). Similarly, a rehabilitation counselor may earn their Certified Rehabilitation Counselor (CRC), and this credential may even be required for them to practice at a state vocational rehabilitation agency. These are voluntary national credentials that are not managed by state organizations. While these voluntary credentials contribute to the counselor's credibility and expertise, they do not necessarily provide oversight to their distance practice. These counselors may be engaging in a distance practice with little oversight. One of the benefits of licensure is oversight by the state regulatory agency, which provides both a standard of excellence for practice (usually including education, experience, and examination), as well as a mechanism for fielding ethical complaints and violations (Gerig, 2018). That being said, some nonlicensed counselors practicing distance counseling may indeed be monitored. Individuals who provide distance counseling as part of their employer services may be overseen by the agency or organization for which they work. For example, school counselors serving students who are home-schooled will likely have similar accountability standards for their distance students as they do for students they serve in a F2F setting. Nevertheless, lack of oversight should be a concern for both the public and the profession.

Credentialing

A license or certification is not a guarantee of counselor competence. While states may not necessarily require a training or certification in DC or TMH, the ACA code (H.1.a.) specifies that practitioners who engage in distance practices have knowledge and skill in relation to their practice. This would indicate that counselors who are engaging in any form of DC and TMH, either from their own practice, their employer's practice, or participating in turnkey platforms, have formalized training in DC and TMH. Training programs do exist; however, the content, cost, and time commitment of these programs vary (Anthony, 2015). The ethical counselor will take the time to research, evaluate and engage in TMH training programs in order to effectively serve their clients and students.

TECHNOLOGY

The lifeblood of DC/TMH is the technology that facilitates its delivery. Distance and TMH modalities may include telephone, text/chat/messaging, video conferencing, and email. Perhaps the biggest challenge for any professional counselor considering distance practice is uncertainty on the technological requirements to practice ethically. While codes provide some guidance, the counselor is often left to determine the specifics of their practice on their own.

Safety and Risk

The wide use of technology in our day to day functioning creates a "false sense of security" among counselors and the general public (Sobelman & Santopietro, 2018, p. 14). News headlines about computer hackers, security breaches, and victims of identity theft may seem like someone else's problems, unless they've happened to someone known to us. Counselors providing DC/TMH services risk not only their own safety and security, but also that of their clients. Monitoring safety and risk includes monitoring physical controls, administrative controls, and technical controls (Sobelman & Santopietro, 2018, p. 15). Physical controls refer to physical safeguards such as locking filing cabinets, locking doors, using security cameras, and other tools that keep the workspace free from intruders or those looking to take information. Administrative procedures include items such as sign-in protocols, policies and procedures manuals, emergency management plans, and screening systems. These systems seek to minimize human error. Finally, technical controls include safety precautions pertaining to technology, including using password protections on devices, firewalls, virus scanning software, and encryption. It is recommended that DC/TMH counselors engage in a formal risk assessment of each area, prior to beginning their practice (Luxton et al., 2016).

Encryption and Privacy

The process of encryption changes plain text to cipher text, with the goal of preventing anyone but the intended party from receiving or interpreting the information (U.S. Department of Commerce, n.d.). Encryption is a security measure that seeks to protect confidential information of the client through transmitted messages, communication, or stored files (Huggins, 2016). Counselors use encrypted devices in order to prevent unauthorized parties from accessing information. Software must also have end-to-end (inaccessible by any third party) encryption, including messaging, email, and video conferencing software. NBCC Standard 5 states that counselors must use secure and encrypted technology, and should explain these security procedures, as well as risks, to clients utilizing DC (NBCC, 2016). For example, during the COVID-19 pandemic, many professional organizations in and beyond the field of counseling began to use the free platform Zoom© for videoconferencing services. Within weeks the platform was circumvented by individuals hacking in to personal meetings and posting inappropriate or unrelated content, known as "zoom-bombing." While Zoom quickly made adaptations and upgrades to their software to correct the concerns (Singer et al., 2020), this example illustrates the potential privacy breeches that can develop, particularly when software that is not designed for counseling or confidentiality is used for such purposes. Counselors must be vigilant about software updates and how those updates may impact the security of client information.

Counselors seek to maintain the confidentiality and privacy of client records. This includes both the storage of and transmission of records or information. Systems used to store, send, or receive client information must be secure. When transmitting information electronically to insurance providers, referrals, or other individuals, the counselor must engage in practices that are HIPAA compliant and protect the ePHI of the client. NBCC (2016) requires that counselors retain copies of written communication delivered via distance formats (Standard 18), and retain service records for 5 years or more depending on state law (Standard 19).

Business Associate Agreements and Third-Party Vendors

Business associates are third-party entities that enhance a counselor's practice by providing a service (Sobelman & Santopietro, 2018). Business associates may include lawyers or accountants, but also include third-party vendors who provide the software and technology for DC/TMH sessions. Counselors must request a written Business Associate Agreement (BAA) from any third-party vendor that they are using for their digital practice, as required by HIPAA. This may include email and videoconferencing software but also electronic medical record (EMR) systems or other file management systems. According to Luxton et al. (2016), "clinical care can easily be addressed by purchasing technology or related connectivity services through reputable vendors who give Business Associate Agreements" (BAA, p. 20). It should be noted that, even with a BAA, when there is a confidentiality breech or violation with the software, the counselor or practice is usually still liable, not necessarily the software provider (Luxton et al., 2016). Requesting and verifying a BAA demonstrates best practices on the part of the counselor, and demonstrates that the counselor followed recommended protocols prior to the violation.

Client Technology

While the counselor may take multiple precautions to ensure the safety and security of client information, there is no assurance that clients will take similar precautions. Counselors are encouraged to educate clients on precautionary measures, such as password protections, encrypted devices, and data security measures, though there is no assurance that the client will adhere to these measures. For this reason, counselors document how and when this information was covered with the client in accordance with ethical practice.

Voice Assistant Technologies

Apple's Siri, Amazon's Alexa, Google Assistant, talk-to-text software, and smart watches are all examples of voice assistant technologies that are common in everyday use. Some people have had a conversation with someone only to realize later it was recorded on a smartphone or smartwatch in talk-to-text. Later these individuals may have discovered advertisements for items discussed during conversations. These are examples of how voice assisted technologies "listen" without being prompted with words such as "Siri," "Alexa," and "Hey Google." Until recently, Apple and Amazon were hiring people to listen to these voice recordings and review the voice transcription quality. Employees reported hearing personal and possibly illegal activities of unknowing consumers, prompting both Amazon and Apple to cease the process and Google to allow an opt-out opportunity for consumers (Denham & Greene, 2019).

Similar concerns exist with listening devices in counseling sessions, whether those sessions be F2F or distance sessions. In both circumstances, the counselor can request that the client put their phone on "airplane mode," disable the listening feature, or turn off the device during session. If the session is F2F or video conference, the counselor can show the client that they are doing the same with their own device. The counselor can request the client show that their phone has been disabled as well. In telephone sessions, the counselor cannot confirm that the client has disabled their listening features. When clients use their mobile devices for telephone or videoconferencing sessions, they are unable to put the phone on airplane mode or turn it off, since a mobile device with Internet connection is most likely needed to conduct the session. Clients can deactivate the listening feature prior to the phone or video session, but again, the counselor is unable to confirm if the client has done so.

It is recommended that counselors disclose these risks to clients prior to conducting sessions and provide detailed instructions to clients on how to deactivate listening modes (Arcuri Sanders, 2020). During F2F sessions, counselors have some control over which devices are in the room during session, based on their physical access to the counseling space. During distance sessions, counselors can request that clients turn off or deactivate the listening features of any voice activated device, but they have little control over how or if that is actually done. As with encryption and other security features, distance counselors can document their requests and policies, as well as include them in their informed consent documents.

CHALLENGES AND OPPORTUNITIES

The benefits of DC and TMH undoubtedly come with some risk. While ethical codes and best practices provide some protection, it's impossible to predict every potential problem in DC and TMH when technology is changing faster than most can keep up.

Duty to Warn

Every counselor is familiar with the concept of "duty to warn"—the need to notify authorities in the event that a student or client is believed to be a danger to themselves or others. In these situations, counselors are trained to seek professional assistance in order to keep the client/others safe, and if needed, contact emergency personnel. The counselor's duty to warn remains when conducting sessions via distance modalities, but the ability to seek assistance or contact emergency personnel is more complex. There are several challenges when a client, located several miles or several hundred miles away from the counselor, expresses intent harm to self or others. Counselors may be unfamiliar with emergency services in the client's area. The counselor may not know where the client is physically located at the time of the call/session. Clients may abruptly end or terminate the session after expressing dangerous intent, and the counselor may be unable to reach them again after they have terminated the session. While all of these situations sound alarming to the counselor considering distance practice, most can be mitigated with proper planning and preparation prior to engaging in DC.

The process begins with a thorough informed consent document outlining the expectations of engaging in distance practice. The ATA (2013) states that informed consents must be reviewed with the client in real time. The ATA also indicates that if signatures are required, electronic signatures are permitted. Specifically, the informed consent should outline the need for emergency information, collateral contacts (referred to as Patient Support Persons by ATA), and emergency personnel in the client's area. It is good protocol to have the client complete an emergency contact (e.g., Patient Support Person) questionnaire, which includes the name of at least two collateral contacts that the client would like contacted in an emergency, also known as an "emergency plan." This plan should include the names and locations of local mental health emergency facilities and the nearest police precinct. If the client will be participating in distance sessions from more than one location (e.g., office and home), then an emergency plan should be created for each location, as the nearest facilities may change based on client location (Luxton et al., 2016). The informed consent should also outline the security measures that will be conducted during each session in order to maintain client safety. These guidelines are reiterated in NBCC Standard 14 (2016).

Clients may desire or elect to conduct sessions in locations beyond those specified on their emergency plans. ATA (2013) recommends discussing with clients who "change locations over the course of treatment" (p. 9) the importance of consistency in treatment locations, as well as the emergency management risks of changing locations. It is also important to note that if the client should relocate out of state, licensure laws and reimbursement policies may be impacted (ATA, 2013). Because of the risk of changing locations, counselors may specify that counseling may only take place in pre-approved locations. In these circumstances, the informed consent should indicate that the counselor will not conduct sessions when the client is at a location other than those with an emergency plan on file. The risk to only allowing sessions in approved locations is that clients may be unwilling to contact counselors in an emergency when not in a designated location.

The counselor should verify the accuracy of information on emergency plans prior to beginning counseling with the client. In the event that the client expresses a danger to themselves or others, counselors can contact the emergency contact indicated on the plan, or if needed, emergency personnel (Luxton et al., 2016). In best case examples, the counselor keeps the client on the phone or video session, while using another device to contact the collateral contact. The counselor can provide the collateral contact with the name of the nearest mental health facility. If the collateral contact cannot or will not escort the client to the nearest mental health facility, emergency personnel can be contacted and dispatched to the client's location.

The protocol described can also be utilized for email, chat, and text sessions, yet these formats are complicated by their asynchronous nature. There is the possibility that a client may express harm to self/others in a message that is not reviewed for hours or days by the counselor. If conducting email/text sessions, it is best to include a statement in the informed consent about delayed counselor response times, not using messaging systems for emergencies, and the expectation to contact 911 or the nearest emergency department in the event of a mental health emergency. Depending on the software used, counselors may be able to send "auto-responses" to incoming messages, which explain the counselor's expected response time and the expectation to contact 911 in an emergency.

A final safety precaution, whether conducting sessions via phone, chat, email or video conference, would be to confirm the location of the client at that moment. This is accomplished simply by asking the client "Where are you located at this time?" The client should be located in a previously designated location in which an emergency plan was created. If the client is not in a previously designated location, the counselor should reference policies outlined in the informed consent document. The ATA (2013) specifies that both the client and counselor share their location, although counselors need not disclose exact addresses if working from a home office. According to the ATA, verification of client and counselor location is critical for four reasons: (a) complying with licensing laws, (b) emergency protocols, (c) mandated reporting, and (d) insurance payment policies.

Confidentiality

Privacy and confidentiality are a concern when conducting TMH and DC. As stated earlier, counselors engage in identity verification in order to ensure that the person they are speaking with is indeed their true client. Yet there are many potential risks to client confidentiality. These include individuals overhearing conversations conducted via phone or video conferencing, particularly when sessions are conducted in the home or in work settings. Similarly, unintended parties may have access to computers, laptops, or devices where clients conduct video, email, text/chat, or phone sessions. Many devices use "auto-save" password features that make it easy for unauthorized individuals to access accounts on shared devices. As discussed earlier, these individuals may attempt to impersonate clients, which is why the use of client verification keywords is critical. NBCC Standard 5 specifies that counselors discourage clients from using auto-save features for passwords. If a client is using laptops or phones that belong to their employer, their employer technically has access to all information on that device (Recupero & Harms, 2016).

Counselors should make every effort to ensure that the client is in a private and confidential location prior to engaging in session. The setting should be free from outside individuals being able to listen or see the session in progress, as well as from potentially distracting activity. In video conference sessions, this is achieved by asking the client to scan the device around the room such that the counselor can see that the setting is private and secure. Similarly, the counselor would also scan their own device around the room to verify for the client that you are speaking from a secure and confidential location. The ATA recommends that if the client is not in a private location, the counselor reviews the risks of conducting session in a non-confidential session (2013). For telephone sessions, counselors verbally confirm that the setting is secure and confidential at the beginning of each call, and also use code words or other identity verification. In an email setting, counselors use code words and password protections to verify identity and minimize potential breaches of confidentiality.

Technology

Technology is growing, changing, and expanding faster than most individuals can follow. Beyond the threats of known individuals accessing client information, TMH is under constant threat of unknown individuals – hackers, scammers, phishers, malware, and other hijackers who seek illegal or unauthorized access to client information. Some of these unknown threats are not necessarily malicious, yet still create risks to our service or security, including software glitches, software updates, and technology upgrades.

One of the challenges of TMH and DC is simply staying informed of all of the changes in technology, including potential risks to client information and security. Distance counselors must remain abreast of changes in technology, and also keep up with security updates and features. As stated, some risks can be mitigated by using encryption and eliminating voice assisted technology. Others may require the assistance of computer or technology professionals to manage the difficulties encountered in TMH practice. These professionals, as well as upgrades to technology and software, require resources. For individuals conducting TMH within their worksite, these costs are usually covered by the employer. However, for the individual considering beginning their own distance practice, the cost of keeping technology current and functioning should be factored into potential costs. For example, many TMH clinicians keep two separate mobile phones—one for personal use and one for client use.

The bottom line is that technology issues, including dropped calls, slow bandwidth, viruses, outdated software and equipment, impact interactions with clients. The quality of the service clients receive is impacted by the technology through which it's delivered. However, the solution may not be upgrading to the latest cutting-edge technology. If the software you upgrade to is only compatible with users who have the newest version of the iPhone, then you will likely cause difficulties and frustrations for your clients with lesser versions, as well as excluding or losing clients altogether who are unable to access your services. Newer software programs may also have unknown glitches and kinks to be worked out. It is recommended that counselors explore trial versions of technologies whenever possible.

CASE STUDY

Counselor A is a TMH counselor who has a state license and training in DC. The counselor maintains a website that is ADA compliant, has a detailed informed consent document, and has working links to the licensing board and emergency contacts, such as hotlines. Counselor A uses secure and encrypted technology, although the counselor has failed to update the system recently due to costs. Counselor A has noticed some lag times in video sessions, the screen freezing more often, and more dropped calls than in the past. Counselor A conducts most sessions via video conference but also permits clients to call, text or email via secure platforms outside of scheduled appointments.

Counselor A has been working with Client B for approximately 6 months. Client B lives in the same state in which Counselor A is licensed, yet lives approximately 300 miles away, in a very rural part of the state. Counselor A developed an emergency contact plan with Client B to identify emergency contacts and services. Client B pursued counseling due to feelings of depression after a recent break up. The client's depression has been immobilizing at times, but the client has not expressed suicidal intent or ideation. As a result of the depression, Client B missed several days of work and was terminated by the employer. This loss of income has threatened Client B's housing and Client B has expressed a fear of becoming homeless. Counselor A is unfamiliar with housing or support services in the client's area. When Client B's parent passed away last year, their primary support system was lost. Counselor A moved Client B to a sliding-scale pay structure due to loss of insurance and health coverage.

On a non-session day, Counselor A received an unsolicited text message from Client B that stated "CAN'T COPE. GIVING UP." Counselor A immediately called Client B who answered but sounded despondent, discouraged, and hopeless. Client B explained that an eviction notice was delivered today and Client B didn't know what to do. Counselor A requested that they transition to a video session and Client B agreed. Once on the video screen, Counselor A could see that Client B was disheveled, distraught, and appeared to be clutching a bottle of medication. When asked about the bottle, Client B disclosed that they had saved a bottle of the parent's pain medication "just in case." Client B was going through the parent's belongings today, thinking about having to move out, and was overwhelmed by how strong the need "to see my parents again" was. At this point, the video session screen appears to lag and before long, the call disconnects. Per the informed consent protocol, Counselor A attempts to reconnect with Client B but is unable to do so via video conference. Counselor A follows protocol and attempts to reach the client via phone and text but the client does not respond to any attempts.

DISCUSSION QUESTIONS

1.   What possible ethics violations or concerns do you note in the case?

2.   How do you feel about using multiple modalities (e.g., text, phone) to reach or assist clients? How was using multiple modalities an asset or a liability in this situation?

3.   The emergency plan states that if the client expresses an intent to harm self or others, emergency contacts will be notified. Counselor A did not have an opportunity to conduct an assessment for lethality. How might that impact your next steps?

4.   If you were Counselor A, would you notify emergency contacts? Would there be any risk that you violated client confidentiality?

5.   Assuming good intent, what did Counselor A do well?

CRITICAL QUESTIONS IN DECIDING TO PRACTICE

In this chapter, we addressed the ethical issues that may impact the practice of TMH and DC. As you consider engaging in a distance practice, reflect on the questions that follow and how they influence your decision to engage in TMH or DC.

1. What is your training in DC and TMH? To what extent are you willing to pursue training and/or certification in this area?
2. How are your technological skills? How skilled are you with smart phones, video conferencing, web-based systems, email and messaging systems?
3. How well would you be able to assess someone else's technology skills? How would you assess client/student appropriateness for DC?
4. What type of investments are you willing to make in technology for your practice? How will you research technologies and keep your technology current? Are you willing to invest in regular upgrades to your technology?
5. What are the laws in your state on TMH pertaining to your license? How will you stay current on these laws? Will the insurance panels you are on reimburse for TMH?
6. If not licensed, what does your national certification indicate about distance practice?
7. How is your attention to detail? What is your ability to create a detailed informed consent document, client verification procedures, and social media policy in order to ensure ethical compliance?
8. Reflect on your social media activity. Are you willing to create separate social media accounts for your practice? Can you commit to maintaining boundaries on social media and avoiding client searches/disclosures?
9. Consider confidentiality. How would you ensure that you engage in secure and confidential practices? What efforts would you take to ensure your clients do the same?
10. Consider your duty to warn responsibilities. How would you manage or navigate a long-distance crisis? What steps would you put in place to ensure that you can best protect your client without violating their confidentiality?

VOICES FROM THE FIELD

Starting Out: What I Wish I Knew Before Diving In

Kellyanne Brady, PhD, LMHC, NCC

When I decided to begin practicing distance counseling, I had very little knowledge of what distance counseling really was. I wanted to gain experience, but before I could do that, I needed to learn about distance counseling. Taking some time to learn about distance counseling before starting was the best thing that I could have done. Not only was it important for me to understand what goes into the process of distance counseling, but it also prepared me for some legal and ethical considerations that were important for me to know from the start. After maintaining an online practice with a large telehealth company and starting my own online practice, I have learned a great deal about the nuances of distance counseling that I never could have learned from the material I was reading before starting.

The first lesson that I learned fairly quickly was boundaries. It's hard to describe that feeling I had when I received my first clients. I was so eager to jump in and get started. There was a mix of excitement and nerves. I was utilizing every feature available through the platform and responding to new clients as quickly as I could. What I didn't realize was that I was setting myself up to get overwhelmed. Before I started, I remember reading that it would be beneficial to only take on one client at a time in order to not overwhelm yourself. Needless to say, I didn't listen. After the first few clients came in, I found myself having difficulty keeping up with the messages and separating "working time" from personal time.

This brings me to the second important lesson I learned, which is the importance of personal limit setting. I started to find that there was never really a time where I wasn't working, and this was challenging for me on several levels. Despite my engagement and excitement, I was burning out. I began to feel stressed and tired more often, and I realized that it was because I never allowed myself the opportunity to "take off." I started to set specific times for working and personal time. I worked hard on developing effective time-management strategies and found strategies to offset the feelings of burnout, which included regular exercise, reading, and practicing mindfulness and stress-reduction exercises.

In addition to the challenge of separating my time, I was also experiencing a blurring of physical boundaries. Something that came as quite a shock to me was the lack of physical separation from my work-life and home-life. Working out of a home office, I found that my home was now the place where I was hearing very difficult stories from clients. Although not really true, I started to feel like there was no escape. I had to develop physical boundaries. I started to ensure that I only worked when inside my home office; not while relaxing on the couch in the living room, or spending time with family. By setting up these physical boundaries, I was then able to practice exercises that helped me separate my time. I made it a point to take breaks to go outside between clients and engage activities that got me away from my computer. By being able to contain the work within the walls of my office, I was able to develop a positive space within the rest of my home; a space where I could reinforce the need for separation from work in order to maintain my own positive mental well-being.

CONCLUSION

Professional ethics is the foundation of counseling practice, and DC and TMHcounseling are no different. A variety of ethical codes exist to guide the professional counselor in their DC/TMH practice, beginning with the ACA and the NBCC. Key elements of these codes address counselor competence, telemental health laws, informed consent, client verification, client relationship, record keeping, and social media. Licensure laws impact the practice of licensed counselors; however, non-licensed counseling professionals also have a responsibility to be appropriately trained and follow ethical guidelines. Counselors must understand the appropriate use of technology in their counseling practice, and be able to assist their clients to understand safety and risks of technology, encryption and privacy, and the use of third-party vendors. Counselors must also be aware of their clients' access to technology, and how the use of voice-assisted technologies may pose risks to confidentiality and security. Two of the greatest challenges counselors face in DC/TMH interventions include duty to warn and risks to confidentiality. Counselors address these risks with proactive planning and reviewing these plans in advance with clients through detailed informed consent documents.

REFERENCES

Acuri Sanders, N. M. (2020, January 14). Hey Siri: Did you break confidentiality or did I? *Counseling Today.* https://ct.counseling.org/2020/01/hey-siri-did-you-break-confidentiality-or-did-i

American Counseling Association. (n.d.). *About us.* https://www.counseling.org/about-us/about-aca

American Counseling Association. (2014). *2014 ACA code of ethics.* https://www.counseling.org/Resources/aca-code-of-ethics.pdf

American Counseling Association. (2020). *Licensure and certification – State professional counselor licensure boards.* https://www.counseling.org/knowledge-center/licensure-requirements/state-professional-counselor-licensure-boards

America's Health Insurance Plans. (2020, April). *Answering the call: Health insurance providers act swiftly as part of the COVID-19 solution.* https://www.ahip.org/wp-content/uploads/Health-Insurance-Providers-Act-Swiftly-as-Part-of-the-COVID-19-Solution.pdf

American Telemedicine Association. (2013, May). *Practice guidelines for video based online mental health services.* https://www.integration.samhsa.gov/operations-administration/practice-guidelines-for-video-based-online-mental-health-services_ata_5_29_13.pdf

Anthony, K. (2015). Training therapists to work effectively online and offline within digital culture. *British Journal of Guidance & Counselling, 43*(1), 36–42, http://dx.doi.org/10.1080/03069885.2014.924617

Baird, M. B., Whitney, L., & Caedo, C. E. (2018). Experiences and attitudes among psychiatric mental health advanced practice nurses in the use of telemental health: Results of an online survey. *Journal of the American Psychiatric Nurses Association, 24*(3), 235–240. https://doi.org/10.1177/1078390317717330

Bloom, J. W. (1997). Guidelines for the new world of webcounseling. *NBCC News Notes, 14*(2). https://www.nbcc.org/Assets/Newsletter/Issues/fall97.pdf

Cipoletta, S., & Mocellin, D. (2018). Online counseling: An exploratory survey of Italian psychologists' attitudes toward new ways of interaction. *Psychotherapy Research, 28,* 909–924. https://doi.org/10.1080/10503307.2016.1259533

Denham, H., & Green, J. (2019, August 2). Did you say "Hey Siri"? Apple and Amazon curtain human review of voice recordings. *The Washington Post.* https://www.washingtonpost.com/technology/2019/08/02/apple-says-its-contractors-will-stop-listening-users-through-siri

Dryman, M. T., McTeague, L. M., Olino, T. M., & Heimberg, R. G. (2017). Evaluation of an open-access CBT-based internet program for social anxiety: Patterns of use, retention, and outcomes. *Journal of Consulting & Clinical Psychology, 85,* 988–1000. https://doi.org/10.1037/ccp0000232

Epstein Becker Green Law. (2020). *Telemental health laws update.* https://www.ebglaw.com/covid-19-telemental-health-laws-update/

Epstein Becker Green Law. (2019). *Telemental Health Laws [mobile application software].* https://play.google.com/store

Gerig, M. S. (2018). *Foundations for clinical mental health counseling: An introduction to the profession* (3rd ed.). Pearson.

Imig, A. (2014). Small but mighty: Perspectives of rural mental health counselors. *The Professional Counselor, 4,* 404–412. https://doi.org/10.15241/aii.4.4.404

Health Resources and Services Administration. (2019, August 16). *Shortage areas.* https://data.hrsa.gov/topics/health-workforce/shortage-areas

Huggins, R. (2016). Using mobile phone communication for therapeutic intervention. In S. Goss., K. Anthony., L. Sykes Stretch, & D. Merz Nagel (Eds.), *Technology in mental health: Applications in practice, supervision, and training* (2nd ed). Charles C. Thomas Publishing.

Kaplan, D. M., Francis, P. C., Hermann, M. A., Baca, J. V., Goodnough, G. E., Hodges, S., Spurgeon, S. L., & Wade, M. E. (2015). New concepts in the *ACA*

Code of Ethics. Journal of Counseling & Development, 95, 110–120. https://doi. org/10.1002/jcad.12122

Luxton, D. D., Nelson, E. L., & Maheu, M. M. (2016). *A practitioner's guide to telemental health: How to conduct legal, ethical, and evidence-based telepractice.* American Psychological Association.

National Board of Certified Counselors. (2016). *Policy regarding the provision of distance professional services.* https://www.nbcc.org/Assets/Ethics/ NBCCPolicyRegardingPracticeofDistanceCounselingBoard.pdf

Recupero, P. R., & Harms, S. (2016). Using email to conduct a therapeutic relationship. In S. Goss., K. Anthony., L. Sykes Stretch, & D. Merz Nagel (Eds.), *Technology in mental health: Applications in practice, supervision, and training* (2nd ed). Charles C. Thomas Publishing.

Singer, N., Perlroth, N., & Krolik, A. (2020, April 8). Zoom rushes to improve privacy for consumers flooding its service. *New York Times.* https://www.nytimes. com/2020/04/08/business/zoom-video-privacy-security-coronavirus.html

Sobelman, S. A., & Santopietro, J. M. (2018). Managing risk: Aligning technology use with the law, ethics codes, and practice standards. In J. J. Magnavita (Ed.) *Using technology in mental health practice.* American Psychological Association.

U.S. Department of Commerce's National Institutes for Standards of Technology. (n.d.). *Computer security resource center: Glossary (encryption).* https://csrc.nist. gov/glossary/term/encryption

U.S. Department of Justice, Civil Rights Division. (2003). Web accessibility under Title II of the ADA. *ADA Best Practices Toolkit for State and Local Government.* https://www.ada.gov/pcatoolkit/chap5toolkit.htm

Zur, O. (2019). *Professional association codes of ethics and guidelines on telemental health, e-therapy, digital ethics, and social media.* https://www.zurinstitute.com/ ethics-of-telehealth/#top

4

Psychosocial and Multicultural Development

INTRODUCTION

There is no doubt that the growth of technology and the emergence of the Internet has had tremendous impact on the human race. Along with advances in science and medicine, the advances in technology and the development of the Internet have shaped many human interactions in ways not previously imagined possible, including counseling interactions. From these developments emerged the concepts of telehealth, telemental health (TMH) and distance counseling (DC). The benefits that technology and the Internet have created for the human race are innumerable, including limitless access to information and the ability to connect with others at great distances. However, among these benefits, there are also difficulties, challenges, and dangers. The birth of the Internet and mobile technology spawned concepts such as cyber bullying, cyber stalking, cyber sexual assault, and other traumas. The Internet allows one to send and receive information almost instantaneously. Yet these transmissions include information that is both accurate and inaccurate, helpful and injurious. All of these elements—good and bad—impact human development. Additionally, the use of technology is not evenly distributed or equitably utilized among diverse populations. This chapter addresses both the developmental and cultural issues that technology brings to the DC/TMH environment, and the counselor's responsibility to address these issues in concert with ethical treatment.

IMPACT OF TECHNOLOGY ON HUMAN DEVELOPMENT

Most theories of human development, including those of Piaget, Erikson, and others, were developed before the emergence of modern technology or in the early stages of its development. Some have argued that since these theories did not initially consider technology, the profession should seek opportunities to connect technology to these theoretical foundations (Pea & Cole, 2019). The definition of technology itself has changed. "For the Ancient Greeks, a technology combined two linked features: *techne*—an art or craft, and *technologia*—the systematic treatment of such arts and crafts" (Pea & Cole, 2019, p. 15). Presently, we consider technology to include not only the technological devices (e.g., hardware, computers, tablets, smart phones, smart watches), but also technological systems (e.g., software, Internet, social media, texting, email) and technological outcomes (e.g., papers, spreadsheets, presentations, videos, pictures, images, messages, memes). These technological concepts impact human development throughout the lifespan.

Human Development

As human beings grow, they develop cognitively, emotionally, socially, and morally, as well as physically. As previously discussed, the use of technology impacts nearly every area of human interaction. Technology plays a role in **cognitive development**, specifically in relation to learning. This includes both the traditional classroom and the homeschooled or remote learning environments that were forced by the COVID-19 crisis. Yet how exactly does digital learning impact cognitive development? In relation to brain activity, learning and complex thinking occur in the neocortex. During periods of intense emotion, the amygdala takes over (Globokar, 2018). Digital learning creates an emotional response in the amygdala, which engages learners, yet detracts from the complex thinking occurring in the neocortex. Many people believe that technology fosters their ability to multitask, claiming that they can listen to music, watch movies, search the web, send email, and engage in a multitude of tasks due to the ease and accessibility of technology (Courage et al., 2015). However, when people multitask, they aren't able to intently focus on one activity, which may explain why students who multitask sometimes earn poorer grades than those who focus on one activity at a time (Courage et al., 2015; Globokar, 2018). Children, adolescents, and adults who experience multiple stimuli from various technological sources may struggle with issues, such as focus, concentration, complex decision-making, and abstract thought.

Technology impacts concepts of **moral development** such as patience, empathy, and kindness. Technology often provides instant gratification and immediate feedback. The human race appears to have grown impatient with waiting. Life lessons such as learning to be patient, taking turns, or having to wait for something that is desired are important skills for human beings; life doesn't happen with the push of a button (Globokar, 2018). Others fear that characteristics such as empathy and kindness are lost behind a keyboard, where the senders and receivers of messages often appear to be anonymous. The media provides many examples of insensitive, cruel, or hurtful ways people have used technology to harm one another. A college student uses a webcam to expose a roommate's sexual orientation; the roommate dies by suicide after learning of the recording; the student is charged with a hate crime (Parker, 2012). A boy texts his girlfriend expressing a desire to die by suicide; her response texts encourage him to complete the act; the boy dies by suicide; the girlfriend is charged with involuntary manslaughter (Levenson et al., 2020). A social media group is created for an incoming class of students to a prestigious Ivy League university; members of this group post racially and sexually offensive images to the group; ten incoming freshman have their admissions offers rescinded as a result of their behavior (Natanson, 2017). There is no shortage of ways people have used technology to cause harm. On the other side of the coin, however, are the online charities and positive viral messages that have been created through technology. People have found creative ways to use technology to help one another, including online fundraising, organizing donation drives, raising awareness, or creating apps that do everything from organizing meals for a family in need to providing sight assistance to the visually impaired.

An individual's **social development** requires that one grows and interacts with other children and adults. Individuals use these interactions to make sense of the outside world, and their own place within that world. Technology has been praised for its ability to bring people together through tools such as email, videoconferencing, chatting, texting, and social media. Affinity groups and interest groups allow people to connect with others who share their passions and concerns, or connect with others at great distances. Despite these connections, there is ample evidence that exclusionary behavior, cyber bullying, and cyber stalking are rampant. There is evidence that some technology, specifically social media, may be contributing to child, adolescent, and adult loneliness (Barth, 2015; Globokar, 2018). Globokar (2018) points out the incongruence between society's value of autonomy, independence, and being unique, in comparison to online society's reliance on "likes" and approval from others.

There is also the issue of people's online personae varying from their true personae. While this is not problematic in and of itself, conflicts arise when people compare their own lives to those of their social connections.

Specifically, individuals evaluate the life activities, social outings, and body images of others, without awareness or understanding that these postings may have been fabricated or altered for the online community. These comparisons can impact the emotional wellness of adolescents and adults alike.

The use of social media has been both praised and criticized for its impact on the emotional development of adolescents. According to Barth (2015), "many, if not all of the normal developmental dynamics, conflicts and stages of contemporary adolescence are experienced through social media and cyber technology" (p. 207). One conflict of contemporary adolescence is bullying, which has morphed into cyberbullying in this technological age. Unlike traditional bullying, cyberbullying takes place inside and outside of the school setting, and the individual may be exposed to constant bullying 24/7 through technological devices such as social medial and mobile phones.

The Cyberbullying Research Center (2019) provides a glossary of over 100 definitions and terms that are used to clarify the understanding and scope of cyberbullying. A sample of selected terms include cyberbullying, cyberstalking, and cyberthreats. While these terms may be self-explanatory, other language is less intuitive, including words such as "fabotage" where a user pretends to be someone else on Facebook; "flaming" or "griefing" which describes sending harassing messages to people privately, in a group, or during a game; "grooming" used to describe adults' attempts to connect with children via the Internet; and "Revenge Porn" or "sextortion" which is used to describe sending intimate photos (or threatening to do so) without someone's consent (Hinduja & Patchin, 2019, pp. 2–5). These definitions provide context for the potential emotional harm that social media and other technologies create. Conversely, there is evidence to suggest that when individuals are in emotional distress, they may reach out for help via technology due to the seemingly anonymous nature of tools, such as text lines, hotlines, or chat sessions (Miller, 2016).

Concerns in relation to adolescent sexual development have increased with Internet use. It is believed that adolescents are receiving information about sexual practices via pornography viewed on the Internet. Pornography often presents images that objectify women and sensationalizes sexual behavior, while also promoting promiscuity, sexual violence, and a distorted view of sexual encounters (Tylka & Cook-Cottone, 2016). Through technology, the pornography industry has expanded to include interactive digital sex through avatars and virtual reality (VR). For some individuals, this use of digital sexual activity, termed "digisexualities," is primary to their sexual identity (McArthur & Twist, 2017, p. 335). This movement away from passive observation of pornography, toward engaging in interactive digital sexual behavior, may be unfamiliar to many professional counselors. McArthur and Twist (2017) explain that with the emergence of technology and the ability to personalize digital robots, the use of digital technology may become an individual's primary source of sexual activity. Counselors will need to be prepared to address these behaviors clinically, without stigma, and without pathologizing them unnecessarily.

Physical health and wellness are part of an individual's physical development. Parents and doctors have expressed concern about the amount of "screen time" children and adolescents partake in daily. There have been fears that sedentary, screen-time behavior will lead to obesity, eye strain, irritability, and problematic sleep patterns. The American Academy of Pediatrics (AAP) recommends avoiding digital media for children below ages 18 to 24 months. Other recommendations include: limiting use to 1 hour per day for children ages 2 to 5 years, not using technology to calm children, no screen-time 1 hour before bed, and building in nonscreen play time (AAP, 2016). However, as children age to adolescence and adulthood, technology use becomes almost essential. Most adults and adolescents have used the Internet to search for medical or physical health information. Many have "Googled" their symptoms, a medication they were prescribed, or cures for ailments. While reputable information can be found, there are concerns that these searches produce advertisements and product placement. In addition, there is worry that adolescents are locating information that is damaging to their physical health, such as food restriction, starving, purging, and body hatred techniques (Tylka & Cook-Cottone, 2016). Other risky behaviors include the ability to purchase medication, vapes, and illicit substances via the Internet.

Physical development also includes aging. There is often a misconception that older adults cannot use technology or are unable to use technology. In studies of older adult computer use, findings indicate that an overwhelming majority of individuals aged 58 to 84 had a computer and Internet access in their homes, whereas less than half of those 85 to 95 years old reported having computer access. Non-use was more likely to be affiliated with age (over 74), gender (female), lower educational level, and being unemployed, as well as being widowed (Siren & Knudsen, 2016). Most older adults tended to balance the benefits and usefulness of computers with the perceived downside of losing personal contacts. The use of computers in employment positively impact older adults' computer use, indicating there may be limited motivation to learn new technologies outside of a work setting (Hargittai & Dobransky, 2017).

Parent and Child Relations

There have been criticisms of technology seemingly taking over the roles of parenting and child care. Conversely, technology has been praised for interactive learning and engaging children in learning concepts. Parents of toddlers 18 to 24 months old were surveyed on use of technology with their children (Gunuc & Atli, 2018). Parental reasons for such use of technology included keeping the child focused while eating or while the parent was conducting other tasks. Parents also reported using technology to make their child happy or to calm down an upset child, yet they also agreed that children became distressed when the technology was removed or when the parent attempted to take it away. Parents also believed that using the technological learning programs enhanced children's language and learning. However, some research suggests that digital learning removes the natural learning that occurs when children observe and attempt behavior via trial and error (Gunuc & Atli, 2018).

The use of technology can bring stress to a household for both children and parents. Studies show that parents feel pressure to introduce their children to technology at a young age in order to remain current with education and social trends (Radesky et al., 2016). Parents of children ages 0 to 8 years expressed worry that not using technology will put their children at a disadvantage in school or society. Parents also believed that online educational learning tools helped their children feel independent. Parents expressed trust in the product descriptions, and relied mostly on the applications' recommendations or reviews prior to downloading. Parents express fear of losing control of their child's technology use. Technology has been described as "unfamiliar territory, where children knew better than parents how to navigate it" (Radesky et al., 2016, p. 506). Parents also expressed guilt for allowing children to play longer than they would prefer. In a study of tablet use among 8- and 9-year-olds, researchers found that children used tablets primarily for socialization, games, entertainment (films and music), education (homework and reading), as well as "going on the web" (Hadlington et al., 2019, p. 20). Children also reported parental struggles with setting boundaries, using technology to escape, and indicators of dependence on their tablets, including being preoccupied with thoughts of the tablet, uncontrollable urges to use the tablet, and problems turning it off.

Addictive Behavior

There has been growing apprehension about technology dependence and addiction among both parents and mental health providers. Process addictions (PA) include compulsive behaviors, not related to substance use, that include issues of cravings, urges, feelings of pleasure, and disruption of daily functioning in pursuit of the behavior (Carlisle et al., 2016). Gambling disorder was the first PA to appear in the latest version of the *Diagnostic*

Statistical Manual of Mental Disorders, Fifth Edition (DSM-5). Internet addiction (IA), while not a recognized disorder in the *DSM-5*, constitutes elements of addiction, as well as impulse control disorders, which impacts children and adults alike. While the Internet provides individuals with a wide array of information and activities, these activities may lead to addictive behaviors including Internet gaming, pornography, shopping, gambling, sex shopping, and social media (Carlisle et al., 2016). While there are no *DSM-5* diagnostic criteria for Internet addiction, there are standardized assessments. Internet addiction resembles other addictive disorders including compulsive use, inability to stop use, preoccupation with using, adverse social/economic/educational/career impact from use, and neglecting other significant life activities. The Cyberbullying Research Center defines the term **webdrawl**, as "The act or process of going without the use of the Internet which one has become addicted" (Hinduja & Patchin, 2019, p. 6).

TECHNOLOGY AND COMMUNICATION

The first web browser appeared in 1993 at the National Center for Supercomputing Applications, after a series of Internet applications dating back to the 1960s and 1970s (Pea & Cole, 2019). Around the turn of the 21st century, Pea and Cole define a "multidimensional explosion" (2019, p. 25) in which digital media saw rapid growth and development. This development included (a) technology moving faster, being cheaper, and usable on smaller devices with more connectivity; (b) "ubiquitous connectivity" (p. 25) in which we became globally connected through trillions of devices; and (c) the richness of the media moved beyond alpha-numeric text to include graphics, audio, video, 3D images, avatars, and artificial intelligence. The immersion of connectivity and information impacts the way individuals communicate with one another. An example of this digital communication is DC/TMH, where the technology facilitates the communication between client and counselor.

Millennials, considered to be individuals born from the mid-90s to the early 2000s, are often said to be digital natives. The term *digital natives*, coined by Marc Prensky (2001), describes a group of individuals who have never known a life without technology. This group of has always had access to the broadband Internet, mobile phones, video games, email, texting, and related technology. For digital natives, the use of technology for communication is natural, if not preferred, to face-to-face communication. In Prensky's words,

> Digital Natives are used to receiving information really fast. They like to parallel process and multi-task. They prefer their graphics before their text rather than the opposite. They prefer random access (like hypertext).

They function best when networked. They thrive on instant gratification and frequent rewards. (2001, para. 11)

Digital immigrants, on the other hand, have had to learn technology. Digital immigrants likely used hard wired phones before mobile phones, typewriters and word processors before computers and tablets, paper maps before GPS systems, cassette tapes before downloads, and countless other examples. According to Prensky, digital immigrants will acculturate to technology at different rates, with some learning and adapting quickly, while others struggle to use the new technology.

The professional counselor engaging in DC/TMH may be either a digital native or a digital immigrant. Many professional counselors would qualify as millennials and digital natives. Technology may be interwoven into their daily lives, including work, school, and their personal lives. Their counseling training may have included information on DC/TMH; these counselors likely made digital recordings of their counseling sessions that were sent electronically to their supervisors during their training. In contrast, other professional counselors may be digital immigrants. These counselors remember recording their counseling sessions on full-size VHS tapes during graduate school, which they later viewed on a VCR during supervision. Digital immigrant counselors have had to learn digital technologies and adapt at different levels. For this reason, it is essential that DC/TMH practitioners assess their own comfort and competence with technology prior to engaging in DC/TMH practice.

More importantly, the clients we serve may be digital immigrants or digital natives. They may have known technology their entire lives, or only recently learned technology. This was apparent during the COVID-19 shelter-in-place order, in which counseling services either transitioned to DC/TMH or ceased entirely. In states that enforced work from home orders, both counselors and clients found themselves navigating a new and uncertain world. Digital natives may feel frustrated and confused by the lack of efficient technology use. Digital immigrants may also feel frustrated or embarrassed by their lack of technological understanding.

Counseling using DC/TMH relies on open communication and mutual understanding between client and counselor. It for these reasons that counseling's ethical codes require counselors to assess the client's technical capabilities, and to develop a detailed informed consent outlining expectations (American Counseling Association [ACA], 2014). However, the counselor may also wish to assess technological preferences. For example, many digital natives may prefer a text to a voicemail, whereas a digital immigrant may reserve texting for close friends and family. These discrepancies should be addressed prior to beginning counseling. These discussions are important in order to avoid stereotypes and assumptions. For example, assuming that older clients are not familiar with technology would be unwise, as many older adults, particularly those in the work force, have been using technology successfully for many years. Similarly, assuming that a younger client is comfortable with technology would also be unwise, as socioeconomic differences create a distinction between those with technology and those without.

CULTURAL IMPLICATIONS

Culturally competent counseling practice begins with an assessment and understanding of one's own culture. This self-assessment includes understanding one's worldview, biases, power, and privileges, and considering how one's experiences may impact their counseling practice (Ivey et al., 2018). This same assessment occurs before engaging in DC/TMH practice. It has previously been discussed how DC/TMH allows client access to more diverse counselors, including counselors who possess cultural and linguistic characteristics that meet the client's need. DC/TMH also allows clients to access counselors who have specializations with specific identity groups including rural communities; veterans; persons with disabilities; lesbian, gay, bisexual, transgender, and queer/questioning (LGBTQ) populations; and other cultural groups. Yet despite DC/TMH creating opportunities for access, there are gross disparities among groups that actually have access to and regularly use distance technologies.

Equity and Access to Technology

Like education, income, housing, job opportunities, and health care, access to technology is not equal. While the United States boasts one of the highest connectivity rates for a country its size (World Bank, 2019), there are distinct differences among those who are connected and those who are not. According to a Pew Research study (2019), 90% of all Americans use the Internet. The Internet is used most often by individuals aged 18 to 49 (97%–98%), followed by 88% of those aged 50 to 64, and 73% of those over 65. White Americans account for 92% of Internet users, followed by Hispanic (86%) and Black (85%) users. Women and men use the Internet almost equally (90%–91%). Income also creates disparities, as 98% of households earning $75,000 or more use the Internet, compared to 82% of those earning less than $30,000. Similarly, 98% of college graduates use the Internet, compared to 71% of those with less than a high school diploma. Suburban communities are the most connected communities with 95% Internet access, compared to 91% in urban areas, and 85% of rural areas (Pew Research Center, 2019).

Broadband Internet creates opportunities to access information faster and quicker than standard Internet. The disparities among groups become more pronounced in relation to broadband usage. White users account for 79% of broadband usage, compared to 66% of Blacks and 61% of Hispanics. Households earning $75,000 or more report 92% broadband use compared to 56% of those earning less than $30,000. Similarly, 79% of college graduates use broadband compared to 46% of those with less than a high school diploma. Suburban communities again report the highest rates of broadband use at 79%, compared to 75% in urban areas, and 63% of rural areas (Pew Research Center, 2019).

These inconsistencies demonstrate that all Internet access is not created equal. Thus, while counselors may view DC/TMH services as creating access to diverse populations, not all populations will be able to access the service. These are important considerations when beginning an online practice or suggesting a DC/TMH service to clients and students. In addition to screening for comfort and competence with technology, counselors must also screen for accessibility, noting that limited access may be attributed to socioeconomic, educational, or geographic factors.

Rural Communities

There is ample evidence to suggest that DC/TMH brings much needed counseling services to rural communities, which traditionally suffer from shortage of access to medical providers and mental health providers. TMH in rural communities has been found to reduce wait time, increase access to providers, and increase collaboration (Holland et al., 2018). The use of TMH in rural communities is growing. In a study of Medicare beneficiaries in rural communities, TMH visits increased from 0.2% to 5.3% between 2004 and 2014, with some states such as Iowa and South Dakota reporting TMH accounting for 10% of all visits. Data indicated that some states conducted 25% of all mental health visits via TMH in 2014 (Mehrotra et al., 2017). However, disparities were noted among the increased usage. For example, White participants accounted for over 85% of TMH sessions, compared to 9.3% of Black participants. These discrepancies may be an indication of socioeconomic differences and inequitable access to healthcare. A contributing factor may be negative perceptions of mental health treatment within the Black community (Avent Harris et al., 2020). Other challenges that TMH brings to rural communities are TMH startup costs (Avent Harris et al., 2020; Lambert et al., 2016), and completing required documentation with families to treat children and adolescents (Nelson & Bui, 2010).

Veterans

The mental health and counseling needs of veterans gained attention with reports of increased veteran suicides beginning around 2005 and peaking in 2014 (Veterans Administration, 2019). Increasingly, TMH/DC interventions are being utilized with military populations, with successful outcomes. In a study of veterans with depression that utilized in-home TMH groups and face-to-face (F2F) treatment groups, depressive symptoms decreased significantly among both groups, although greater improvement was noted among F2F groups. While the F2F groups saw greater improvement, "there was not any evidence of clinical worsening in the in-home condition to suggest that in-home care was less safe than traditional in-office care" (Luxton et al., 2016, p. 930). Similarly, TMH has been used with complex clinical issues. In a study of female veterans in rural communities who were victims of military sexual trauma (MST), implementing a TMH intervention was found to significantly reduce symptoms of posttraumatic stress disorder (PTSD) and depression, as well as significantly improve emotional regulation (Weiss et al., 2018). Despite these positive outcomes with TMH interventions, there is evidence to suggest that military veterans may be hesitant to engage in TMH practices. Specifically, those with positive screenings for PTSD were less likely to report a willingness to use TMH interventions (Whealin et al., 2015).

Persons With Disabilities

Another population that may benefit from DC/TMH services are persons with disabilities (PWD). DC/TMH has the capacity to provide counseling access to individuals with limited transportation and limited mobility, which may include PWD. The use of technology for communication is not a new concept among PWD. Prior to the widespread use of DC/TMH, PWD were using technology to communicate through TTY (text telephone) devices, light talkers, smart boards, touch pads, and other augmentative and alternative communication devices. Access to mental health care is often difficult for members of the deaf community, particularly for those who use American Sign Language (ASL), as their primary language. Counselors may mistakenly assume that members of the deaf community would prefer written TMH, yet Crowe (2017) explains that video sessions using ASL would be preferable. "Written correspondence between a hearing provider and patient is often ineffective, especially with those for whom ASL is the primary language and English is a secondary language" (Crowe, 2017, p. 158). For the counselor engaging in DC/TMH with PWD, the focus should be on developing accommodations and adaptations for a successful session.

Lesbian, Gay, Bisexual, Transgender, and Queer/Questioning (LGBTQ)

LGBTQ individuals have benefited from being able to connect to other LGBTQ adults through Internet platforms and social groups (Hutchins, 2013; Singh & Chum, 2013). The ability to find support or conduct research on the Internet can be incredibly valuable for members of the LGBTQ community, their family, friends, and loved ones. Many older members of the LGBTQ community have shared difficulties in finding connections or getting information when growing up in a pre-Internet era. Being able to access information on LGBTQ health concerns is vital for adolescents and adults who may be unable to safely or comfortably ask questions about medical issues in their home or with their primary care provider. Despite these benefits, there are also concerns that Internet relationships may contribute to isolation, alienation, and remaining closeted, particularly among gay men (Hutchins, 2013). One benefit of DC/TMH services to LGBTQ populations is the ability to access counselors who have experience working with LGBTQ clients or concerns. One such service is Pride Counseling (www.pridecounseling.com), which provides DC/TMH services to the LGBTQ population from counselors who are supportive and knowledgeable of LGBTQ issues.

Cultural History

The Internet can provide access to information about individual cultures that has either been washed out of history books or lost among family traditions. In interviews, Tommy Orange, best-selling Native author of the book, *There There* (2018), describes how many Native persons have turned to the Internet to research history, genealogy, and cultural practices of Native communities dispersed by American settlers. Similarly, websites, such as Slave Voyages (www.slavevoyages.org) and African Origins (www.african-origins.org), provide information and historical tracings of slave routes. These websites, funded and populated by researchers from Emory University, the National Endowment for the Humanities, and other prestigious organizations, trace slave routes between Africa and the Americas, and allow searches by names and African countries. Internet searches can produce reputable and historical information on civil rights movements of LGBTQ groups, PWD, and other populations. Thus the Internet can be used as a resource to both clients and counselors to further understand their own cultural background or the backgrounds of those they serve.

CHALLENGES AND OPPORTUNITIES

The use of DC/TMH can create access to counseling for a multitude of populations, yet may also create challenges for some. Wu and Grant (2013) best describe these dilemmas, stating, "Distance counseling via email and videophone works well for some populations but not others. . . . There is a disproportionately negative impact on those who do not have access to technology" (p. 244). While Wu and Grant use this description to describe working with deaf children and hearing family members, their comments accurately capture both the challenges and opportunities of DC/TMH in relation to psychosocial and multicultural concerns. Fortunately, counselors have opportunities to prepare for these interactions, and attempt to mitigate adverse consequences of DC/TMH for diverse populations.

Professional Organizations

Counselors who wish to expand their knowledge of diverse populations and developmental stages have the opportunity to do so via professional organizations. Whether one practices in DC/TMH or F2F format, professional organizations provide information, insight, research, and professional development on a wide variety of counseling populations. The ACA has 18 divisions which represent diverse areas of clinical practice. Divisions pertaining to psychosocial development may include the Association for Child and Adolescent Counseling (ACAC) or the Association for Adult Development and Aging (AADA). Professional organizations that address multicultural issues may include the Association for Multicultural Counseling and Development (AMCD), American Rehabilitation Counseling Association (ARCA), Counselors for Social Justice (CSJ), Military and Government Counseling Association (MGCA), and Society for Sexual, Affectional, Intersex, and Gender Expansive Identities (SAIGE), formerly Association for Lesbian, Gay, Bisexual, and Transgender Issues in Counseling (ALGBTIC).

Ethics

The 2014 ACA Code of Ethics (H.5.d) specifies that counselors engaging in DC/TMH practice consider both multicultural and disability needs. Clients must be able to access information on counselor websites. This includes websites being accessible to persons with disabilities and offering translation capabilities for various languages based on client population (ACA, 2014). While the ACA codes provide foundational ethics for all counselors, many counseling organizations have developed competencies for working with diverse populations. While these competencies are not specifically aimed at DC/TMH approaches, they provide additional guidance for the counselor who aims to practice with diverse populations. These competencies include ALGBTIC Competencies for Counseling LGBQQIA (2012), ALGBTIC Competencies for Counseling Transgender Clients (2009), ARCA Disability-related Counseling Competencies (2019), Competencies for Counseling the Multiracial Population (2015), and the Multicultural and Social Justice Counseling Competencies (2015; ACA, n.d.). The ARCA Disability-related Counseling Competencies directly reference DC/TMH, stating that counselors "Make efforts to ensure the accessibility of technology used for distance counseling, websites, social media sites, software, and computer applications" (Chapin et al., 2018). Reviewing these competencies is an opportunity for DC/TMH counselors to self-assess their knowledge and increase their training prior to practice, if needed.

Human Connection

One challenge of DC/TMH is that there is a physical distance between the client and counselor. While counselors aren't regularly in physical contact with clients during F2F sessions, they are physically present and attentive to their clients. Small gestures, like asking if the temperature is too cold or too hot, offering a glass of water, or encouraging someone to make themselves comfortable, are elements of human connection that are lost to DC/TMH practices. While not necessary for counseling, these small elements build rapport and also break down power dynamics between clients and counselors. There is evidence to suggest that some older adults prefer human interaction (Siren & Knudsen, 2017). Older adults tend to engage in less risk-taking behavior and may have less trust in the Internet as digital immigrants. For these reasons some agencies have implemented in-home counseling for senior citizens who may be confined to their home and unable to attend counseling. Despite these preferences, technological interventions are recommended with elderly populations, for both psychological evaluations and as a means of assessing elder abuse (Bitondo Dyer et al., 2020). DC/TMH can indeed provide valuable service, but the distance format may minimize human connection that some populations may prefer.

Diverse Client/Counselor Interactions

The opportunity for DC/TMH to connect diverse clients to diverse counselors is monumental. As discussed, clients seeking counselors from various cultural groups and with various linguistic abilities can utilize DC/TMH services to access counselors with desired characteristics. However, there is a lack of diverse and/or multilingual counselors in the field. While digital translation services are available, most agree that they are faulty at best. A client whose first language is not English, may be comfortable speaking to a counselor, but may be less comfortable using email, text, or written communication. Additionally, it has been discussed that technology is not distributed equally. In order to access diverse counselors (assuming they exist), clients from diverse background must (a) know that DC/TMH services exist, (b) know how to access and research diverse counselors that provide DC/TMH, (c) have the financial means to access these services, and (d) have the technological capabilities to engage in DC/TMH services. These challenges are multiplied for clients whose first language is not English, those without medical insurance, and those whose culture stigmatizes seeking counseling services. Thus while it is important to praise the opportunities that DC/TMH creates for diverse clients, it is equally important to recognize the individual and systemic barriers that are in place for members of certain cultural and socioeconomic communities. Counselors have a responsibility to advocate for removal of these systemic barriers and the creation of truly equitable access to treatment.

CASE STUDY: PSYCHOLOGICAL DEVELOPMENT AND MULTICULTURAL DEVELOPMENT

Counselor A works as a care manager for a local nonprofit organization. The organization's mission is to "serve the aging members of our community with dignity, pride, and compassion." In the care manager role, Counselor A provides supportive counseling and case management services to elderly members of the community via home visits and telemental health. Counselor A was directed to conduct an intake with Client B, an 85-year-old African American client, and assess the client's eligibility for services. Counselor A attempted to call Client B on multiple occasions, however no one picked up the phone and there was no ability to leave a voicemail. The following week, Counselor A received a call from Adult Child C. Adult Child C is the child of Client B and was calling to inquire why Client B had not been scheduled for an intake. Counselor A explained that several calls were attempted. Adult Child C explained that Client B does not have an answering machine, does not pick up the phone, and does not have a mobile phone. It was explained that Client B lives alone, in a rural community. As a Korean war era veteran, Client B is eligible for medical care from the VA but is unable to access appointments without transportation. Adult Child C expressed concerns that Client B is lonely, depressed, and may be showing signs of dementia, explaining that Client B "really needs someone to talk to—they just sit in that house all day alone—and I can only get over there a couple of days a week."

Counselor A asked if Adult Child C would be able to bring Client B to the office for an intake evaluation, but they were unable to do so due to conflicts with their work schedule. Adult Child C stated that they would tell their parent to pick up the phone at a mutually agreed upon time. Counselor A called Client B at the mutually agreed upon time, and Client B answered the phone. Counselor A explained the purpose of the call and that they needed to ask some questions in order to determine how they could help. Client B regularly asked Counselor A to repeat themselves over the phone, and became frustrated with their inability to hear the counselor. Client B finally stated, "You know what? This is taking too much of my time. I don't need any help. I just need my medicine and a ride to the VA," and hung up the phone. Counselor A attempted to call back but received no answer. Counselor A realized they did not have a phone number for Adult Child C.

1.   Knowing what you know about Counselor A's agency mission and Client B's case, do you believe that Client B would be appropriate for services?

2.   Discuss Client A's communication with Adult Child C. What were the benefits and risks of discussing this case with the client's child?

3.   Consider Client B's skill, ability, and comfort with technology. Consider Client B's access to technology. How would you assess Client B's appropriateness for TMH?

4.   What role do you believe the client's age, race, community, and veteran status would have on counseling treatment, if at all?

5.   Assuming good intent, what did Counselor A do well?

CRITICAL QUESTIONS IN DECIDING TO PRACTICE

This chapter addressed the elements of psychosocial and multicultural development that may be impacted by technology. It also addressed how counselors can be aware of these issues when preparing to work in DC/TMH settings. Following are some questions to consider in relation to psychosocial and multicultural development and a prospective DC/TMH practice.

1. What developmental age and multicultural group do you plan to work with? What is your experience in working with that population, and would DC/TMH be appropriate?

2. Consider the impact of technology on cognitive, moral, social, emotional, sexual, and physical development. How might these elements relate to the population you seek to serve?

3. Consider the myriad of ways that technology can be used to cause developmental harm. How would you assist your clients/students with issues related to technological harm?

4. What are your thoughts on Internet Addiction? How would you assist a parent or a client who's expressed concern about excessive technology use in themselves or others?

5. Reflect on the information you read on digisexualities. How are you prepared to address issues pertaining to digisexuality or clients viewing sexual content on the Internet?

6. Are you a digital native or a digital immigrant? How might that impact your interactions with the clients/students you serve via DC/TMH?

7. Reflect on your own cultural identity and world view. How might your own identity and world view impact your interactions with clients different than yourself?

8. Assess your own cultural competence. How culturally competent are you in F2F sessions? How would that change for DC/TMH practice, if at all?

9. What professional organizations do you belong to? Which might you join? Which organization's competencies may you need to review to enhance your practice?

10. Consider issues of access and equity. Knowing that technology is not evenly distributed, how will you address those inequities, both in your practice and in your community?

VOICES FROM THE FIELD: HUMAN DEVELOPMENT

Using TMH With Children and Adolescents

Elvira Raposo, Second Year Graduate Student, Clinical Mental Health Counseling

My experience with TMH has been brief and directly impacted with the state of emergency related to COVID-19. Prior to the pandemic, I was interning at an outpatient mental health clinic. Due to the pandemic, I had to undergo a crash course of DC and immerse into TMH rather quickly. The population I work with is children and adolescents between the ages of 4 years old and 15 years old. Within my caseload, my clients possess a wide range of insight and motivation. Due to this, there are several pros and cons that I would associate with DC and this particular population.

An important aspect of counseling with my clients was play therapy. Games played a huge role with our interactions in the office. I found that having a game on which the clients can focus their attention while they spoke made them more open and susceptible to sharing their thoughts and feelings. This goes for both my younger clients and my adolescents. The inability to use play therapy as I had in person has been the biggest challenge in my experience with distance therapy. Although it is quickly evolving and there are therapists finding ways to conduct play therapy through different platforms, it has not been an easy task for me to incorporate. I have found myself coming up with more creative ways to engage my clients, whether through verbal games such as "Simon says" or simply having them share important objects they find in their homes that may be of sentimental value. I have found my clients to be responsive to this form of play; however, it is less productive than play in the office with board games and other tools.

One major benefit I have found in TMH with younger clients is their decreasing self-consciousness. With in-person sessions, my clients were reserved and would divert certain conversations. Now with TMH, those same clients have been more receptive to discussing certain topics and have become more talkative without the pressure of being in the office. I would attribute this to the clients being able to choose a comfortable area in their home, and the safety of their environment helping them become more open to therapy. When compared to my adult clients, the children and adolescents made an easier transition to TMH and were more adaptable to the changes they were facing with this new form of therapy.

One unique aspect of working with this population through TMH is their comfort with technology. My younger clients have known technology all of their lives and have a certain connection with devices that my older clients do not. This unique aspect made their transition easier and they showed a higher level of understanding, not only of the technology, but also of how to build a therapeutic alliance from a distance through a device. For anyone considering using TMH with this population, I would say to be creative and understanding. Children and adolescents need some level of understanding and flexibility. You also need to adapt as the counselor and adjust the session in a way that will be engaging for them. In my opinion, this population is a great prospect for TMH, especially with the fun and creative ways people have been able to incorporate play through different platforms.

VOICES FROM THE FIELD: MULTICULTURAL DEVELOPMENT

Rural Telemental Health Counseling

Michael Jones, PhD, LPC-S, NCC, BC-TMH

I currently serve in a private practice setting in rural Arkansas. According to the 2010 U.S. Census data, Arkansas has approximately 3 million people. Arkansas ranks seventh highest in the nation for the poverty rate and 42% of its residents live in rural areas. I am a rural TMH counseling practitioner.

There are pros and cons in working with rural populations. One major pro of working in a rural setting is that clients have a good idea of the type of clinician you are because word of mouth recommendations carry a lot of weight in smaller communities. It is a normal occurrence for me to come in contact with my clients in a public setting. They are more familiar with me because a previous client has most likely referred them to me. This helps me to remember that my reputation in the public eye can affect my practice and the interactions that I have with my current and future clients. This familiarity normally has a positive effect on the ease of building rapport with my clients.

One major con of working in a rural setting is the lack of equity when it comes to technology in the client's home. For practitioners who are in large cities, it is an expectation that your client will have high speed Internet services or access to free WiFi for counseling sessions. According to a 2016 report from the Federal Communication Commission (FCC), nearly 39% of American in rural areas do not have access to high-speed Internet. This becomes problematic when trying to utilize TMH counseling. This puts the clinician in the position of finding suitable Internet service for their clients.

The one unique aspect of doing TMH counseling with this population is the education that clinicians provide to their clients on information privacy. When you live in an area that is not "technology rich," then there is an undertone of distrust for technology. This distrust can be overcome as clinicians provide the vital information their clients need to put them at ease about the use of technology.

My main piece of advice I would share for someone who practices in a rural area is to practice patience with your clients. When things are new it is natural for there to be some hesitation to try a method of service. I believe as your client's trust builds in you then the level of anxiety about using technology will begin to decrease. This makes it a positive environment for both the client and clinician.

CONCLUSION

The overarching impact of technology has greatly benefited our society. Yet technology also impacts the human development of persons throughout their life span, and may impact certain cultural groups differently than others. Technology can impact an individual's cognitive, moral, social, emotional, sexual, and physical development in a multitude of ways, and may impact older adults differently than younger adults. Technology may also impact parent and child relationships, increase stress, and contribute to addictive behaviors, such as Internet addiction, gambling, shopping, and pornography. Digital natives and digital immigrants will respond differently to the use of technology, and will adapt at different rates to technological interventions. While the use of technology is expanding, certain cultural groups are disadvantaged in their access to technology, specifically those from lower socioeconomic groups, those with less education, and those in rural communities. Alternatively, certain groups benefit from the connections that technology provides, including rural populations, military personnel and veterans, persons with disabilities, and members of the LGBTQ community. The Internet has provided a venue for understanding cultural history for groups whose history is commonly silenced. A multitude of professional development organizations, and ethical codes assist the DC/TMH counselor to develop an awareness of these developmental and cultural concerns. While DC/TMH has the ability to connect diverse clients to diverse clinicians, there continues to be a shortage of diverse practitioners, as well as systemic barriers that limit technological access for several populations.

REFERENCES

American Academy of Pediatrics. (2016). Media and young minds. *Pediatrics, 138*, 1–6. https://pediatrics.aappublications.org/content/pediatrics/138/5/e20162591.full.pdf

American Counseling Association. (n.d.). *Competencies.* https://www.counseling.org/knowledge-center/competencies

American Counseling Association. (2014). *2014 ACA code of ethics.* https://www.counseling.org/Resources/aca-code-of-ethics.pdf

Avent Harris, J. R., Crumb, L., Crowe, A., & Garland McKinney, J. (2020). African American's perceptions of mental illness and preferences for treatment. *Journal of Counselor Practice, 11*, 1–33. https://doi.org/10.22229/afa1112020

Barth, F. D. (2015). Social media and adolescent development: Hazards, pitfalls, and opportunities for growth. *Clinical Social Work, 43,* 201–208. https://doi .org/10.1007/s10615-014-0501-6

Bitondo Dyer, C. , Murdock, C., Hiner, J., Haplern, J., & Burnett, J. (2020). Elder mistreatment intervention: Strategies for connecting with diverse and rural populations. *Generations: Journal of the American Society on Aging, 44,* 91–97.

Carlisle, K. L., Carlisle, R. M., Polychronopoulos, G. B., Goodman-Scott, E., & Kirk-Jenkins, A. (2016). Exploring internet addiction as a process disorder. *Journal of Mental Health Counseling, 38,* 170–182. https://doi.org/10.17744/mehc.38.2.07

Chapin, M., McCarthy, H., Shaw, L., Bradham-Cousar, M., Chapman, R., Nosek, M., Peterson, S., Yilmaz, Z., & Ysasi, N. (2018). *Disability-related counseling competencies.* Author.

Courage, M. L., Bakhtiar, A., Fitzpatrick, C., Kenny, S., & Brandeau, K. (2015). Growing up multitasking: The costs and benefits for cognitive development. *Developmental Review, 35,* 5–41. https://doi.org/10.1016/j.dr.2014.12.002

Crowe, T. V. (2017). Is telemental health services a viable alternative to traditional psychotherapy for deaf Individuals? *Community Mental Health Journal, 53,* 154–162. https://doi.org/10.1007/s10597-016-0025-3

Globokar, R. (2018). Impact of digital media on emotional, social and moral development. *Nova Prisutnost, 3,* 545–560. https://doi.org/10.31192/np.16.3.8

Gunuc, S., & Atli, S. (2018). Parents' view on the impact of technology on 18 to 24-month old infants. *Addicta: The Turkish Journal on Addictions, 5,* 205–226. https://doi.org/10.15805/addicta.2017.5.2.0047

Hadlington, L., White, H., & Curtis, S. (2019). "I cannot live without my [tablet]": Children's experiences of using tablet technology within the home. *Computers in Human Behavior, 94,* 19–24. https://doi.org/10.1016/j.chb.2018.12.043

Hargittai, E., & Dobransky, K. (2017). Old dogs, new clicks: Digital inequality in skills and uses among older adults. *Canadian Journal of Communication, 42,* 195–212. http://doi.org/10.22230/cjc2017v42n2a3176

Hinduja, S., & Patchin, J. W. (2019). *Cyberbullying Research Center Glossary. Social media, cyberbullying, and online safety terms to know.* https://cyberbullying.org/ social-media-cyberbullying-online-safety-glossary.pdf

Holland, J., Hatcher, W., & Meares, W. L. (2018). Understanding the implementation of telemental health in rural Mississippi: An exploratory study of using technology to improve health outcomes in impoverished communities. *Journal of Health and Human Services Administration, 41,* 52–86.

Hutchins, A. M. (2013). Counseling gay men. In C. E. Lee (Ed.). *Multicultural issues in counseling: New approaches to diversity* (4th ed.). American Counseling Association.

Ivey, A. E., Ivey, M. B., & Zalaquett, C. P. (2018). *Intentional interviewing and counseling: Facilitating client development in a multicultural society* (9th ed.). Brooks/Cole.

Lambert, D., Gale, J., Hartley, D., Croll, Z., & Hansen, A. (2016). Understanding the business case for telemental health in rural communities. *Journal of Behavioral Health Services & Research, 43,* 366–397. https://doi.org/10.1007/s11414-015 -9490-7

Levenson, E., Hendersen, J., & Sgueglia, K. (2020, January 23). *Michelle Carter, convicted in texting suicide case, released from prison.* CNN. https://www.cnn.com/2020/01/23/us/michelle-carter-text-suicide-release/index.html

Luxton, D. D., Pruitt, L. D., Wagner, A., Smolenski, D. J., Jenkins-Guarnieri, M. A., & Gahm, G. (2016). Home-based telebehavioral health for U.S. military personnel and veterans with depression: A randomized controlled trial. *Journal of Consulting and Clinical Psychology, 84,* 923–934. https://dx.doi.org/10.1037/ccp0000135

McArthur, N., & Twist, M. L. C. (2017). The rise of digisexuality: Therapeutic challenges and possibilities. *Sexual and Relationship Therapy, 32,* 334–344. https://doi.org/10.1080/14681994.2017.1397950

Mehrotra, A., Huskamp, H. A., Souza, J., Uscher-Pines, L., Rose, S., Landon, B. E., Jena, A. B., & Busch, A. B. (2017). Rapid growth in mental health telemedicine among rural Medicare beneficiaries, wide variation across states. *Health Affairs, 36,* 909–917. https://doi.org/10.1377/hlthaff.2016.1461

Miller, D. N. (2016). Preventing adolescent and young adult suicide. In C. L. Juntunen & J. P. Schwartz (Eds.) *Counseling across the lifespan: Prevention and treatment* (2nd ed.). Sage.

Natanson, H. (2017, June 5). Harvard rescinds acceptances for at least ten students for obscene memes. *The Harvard Crimson.* https://www.thecrimson.com/article/2017/6/5/2021-offers-rescinded-memes

Nelson, E., & Bui, T. (2010). Rural telepsychology services for children and adolescents. *Journal of Clinical Psychology: In Session, 65,* 490–501. https://doi.org/10.1002/jclp.20682

Parker, I. (2012, January 30). The story of a suicide: Two college roommates, a web cam, and a tragedy. *The New Yorker.* https://www.newyorker.com/magazine/2012/02/06/the-story-of-a-suicide

Pea, R., & Cole, M. (2019). The living hand of the past: The role of technology in development. *Human Development, 62,* 14–39. https://doi.org/10.1159/000496073

Pew Research Center. (2019, June 12). *Internet/Broadband Fact Sheet.* https://www.pewresearch.org/internet/fact-sheet/internet-broadband

Prensky, M. (2001). *Digital natives, Digital immigrants.* https://www.marcprensky.com/writing/Prensky%20-%20Digital%20Natives,%20Digital%20Immigrants%20-%20Part1.pdf

Radesky, J. S., Eisenberg, S., Kistin, C. J., Gross, J., Block, G., Zuckerman, B., & Silverstein, M. (2016). Overstimulated consumers or next generation learners? Parent tensions about child mobile technology use. *Annals of Family Medicine, 14,* 503–508. https://doi.org/10.1370/afm.1976

Singh, A. A., & Chum, K. Y. S. (2013). Counseling lesbian, bisexual, queer, questioning, and transgender women. In C. E. Lee (Ed.), *Multicultural issues in counseling: New approaches to diversity* (4th ed.). American Counseling Association.

Siren, A., & Knudsen, S. G. (2017). Older adults and emerging digital service delivery: A mixed methods study on information and communications technology use, skills, and attitudes. *Journal of Aging & Social Policy, 29,* 35–50. https://doi.org/10.1080/08959420.2016.1187036

Tylka, T. L., & Cook-Cottone, C. P. (2016). Health disparities and help-seeking behaviors among girls. In C. L. Juntunen & J. P. Schwartz (Eds.), *Counseling across the lifespan: Prevention and treatment* (2nd ed., pp. 165–185). Sage.

Veterans Administration. (2019). *Office of Mental Health and Suicide Prevention.* 2019 National Veteran Suicide Prevention Annual Report. https://www. mentalhealth.va.gov/docs/data-sheets/2019/2019_National_Veteran_Suicide_ Prevention_Annual_Report_508.pdf

Weiss, B. J., Azevedo, K., Webb, K., Gimeno, J., & Cloitre, M. (2018). Telemental health delivery of Skills Training in Affective and Interpersonal Regulation (STAIR) for rural women veterans who have experienced military sexual trauma. *Journal of Traumatic Stress, 31,* 620–625. https://doi.org/10.1002/jts.22305

Whealin, J., Seibert-Hatalsky, L.A., Willet Howell, J., & Tsai, J. (2015). E-mental health preferences of veterans with without probable posttraumatic stress disorder. *The Journal of Rehabilitation Research and Development, 52*(6), 725–738. https://doi.org/10.1682/JRRD.2014.04.0113

World Bank. (2019). *Individuals using the Internet (% of population – United States).* International Technological Union, World Telecommunications/ICT Development report and database. https://data.worldbank.org/indicator/ IT.NET.USER.ZS?locations=US

Wu, C. L., & Grant, N. C. (2013). Counseling deaf children and their hearing families: Working with a constellation of diversities. In C. E. Lee (Ed.). *Multicultural issues in counseling: New approaches to diversity* (4th ed.). American Counseling Association.

5

Individual Counseling and Telemental Health

INTRODUCTION

In the wake of the COVID-19 pandemic, it is possible that hundreds if not thousands of mental health practitioners made the transition to telemental health (TMH) services between March and April of 2020. Simultaneously, school counselors, vocational rehabilitation counselors, career counselors and others transitioned to distance counseling (DC) modalities. These broad sweeping transitions were supported by school systems and state governments. University and K-12 classrooms were converted to distance learning platforms in a matter of weeks, if not days. Departments of education and mental health services scrambled for mechanisms to continue or expand counseling to clients and students via remote practice. The Council on the Accreditation of Counseling and Related Education Programs (CACREP) published a document on flexibility of specific standards regarding practicum and internships (e.g., professional practice). Specifically, CACREP's flexibility standard stated that "CACREP does not have any prohibitions against telemental health or distance supervision" (CACREP, 2020, para. 8), indicating that counseling students may utilize TMH. CACREP did specify that programs "must ensure that students and site supervisors are trained to use this modality" (para. 9).

The transition to TMH/DC was supported by the U.S. Department of Health and Human Services (DHHS) Office of Civil Rights' unprecedented statement on March 17, 2020 indicating that the DHHS "will not impose penalties for noncompliance with the regulatory requirements under the HIPAA [Health Insurance Portability and Accountability Act] Rules against covered health care providers in connection with the good faith provision of telehealth during the COVID-19 nationwide public health emergency" (DHHS, 2020, para. 4). The statement does not allow for reckless practice, and emphasized good faith efforts. Yet many counseling practitioners, including those with little training and experience in DC/TMH, viewed the transition as a good faith effort to meet their clients' needs. While these transitions were indeed designed to help clients and students, HIPAA compliance is only one component of effective and ethical practice. It is possible that counselors and counseling students who transitioned without proper training may have missed the basic fundamentals and logistics of DC/TMH that could have impacted their practice with individual clients.

Prior research has demonstrated that most counselors are dissatisfied with the level of training they received in DC/TMH and express uncertainty on TMH guidelines (Baird et al., 2018; Centore & Milacci, 2008; Perle et al., 2012; Simms et al., 2011). Yet alarmingly, these same studies found that nearly 75% of practitioners who were dissatisfied with their training and had previously engaged in TMH practice (Baird et al., 2018; Centore & Milacci, 2008). In order to avoid future treatment without training, counselors who are committed to providing effective treatment for their clients and students must understand both the logistics and clinical skills required to practice in a distance environment.

LOGISTICS OF INDIVIDUAL PRACTICE

The start of one's DC/TMH practice begins with preparation and ethics. Once a counselor has sufficiently addressed safety precautions, such as informed consent, encrypted technologies, confidentiality, and a safety plan, they can begin to move on to the logistics of DC/TMH practice.

Professional Workspace

Counselors begin by examining the workplace in which they intend to engage in distance practice. The workspace should ensure confidentiality and be free from distractions and outside noise. For synchronous sessions, use of a white noise machine can help with confidentiality and minimize the likelihood of others overhearing client/student conversations. The use of headphones by both the counselor and client will minimize the ability for outside parties to hear conversations and discussions. For video sessions, the setting should be professional, free from clutter and personal artifacts. When conducting DC/TMH in one's home, using an office or a neutral space, as opposed to one's bedroom or kitchen helps to maintain professional boundaries and privacy of the counselor. If using WiFi or mobile devices, counselors should attempt to work in areas that have the strongest, most reliable signal. In some cases, it may be best to use wired Internet or landlines, as opposed to WiFi or mobile phones, if available. A professional workspace also includes the use of secure and encrypted technologies that both the client and counselor are capable of using, as well as a space that is free from voice-recognition software (Arcuri Sanders, 2020).

Distractions

The workspace should be free of distractions. If conducting phone or videoconferencing sessions, turn off other functions on the PC/device in order to minimize interruptions (Kozolowski & Homes, 2017). Distractions, such as incoming emails or notifications, can draw a counselor's attention away from the client. If one were conducting a face-to-face (F2F) session, the counselor would not be looking at emails during the session, and similarly should avoid viewing emails or other functions during DC/TMH sessions. Counselors can minimize distractions by closing other programs. For video sessions, this has the added benefit of improving bandwidth speed and reducing lag time. It is recommended that counselors slide the computer away from themselves and out of arm's length in order to avoid using other computer functions (Kozolowski & Homes, 2017). This also allows the client to see more of the counselor's body language and encourages clients to do the same. Silencing phones that are not being used (e.g., house phones, mobile phones) is another strategy to minimize distractions. Research has also found counselors to be distracted by looking at themselves in their video (Kozolowski & Homes, 2014). If counselors are distracted by their own images, consider minimizing the video image if that is an option with the software being used.

Distractions are less likely when conducting email or text sessions, but possible nonetheless, specifically if using recorded messages (audio or video) for client communication. Some noises and distractions are beyond the counselor's control, such as a doorbell ringing, or a dog barking excessively at the ringing doorbell. Counselors can discuss these potential distractions with clients in advance, take steps to reduce distractions, and keep their focus on the client should these distractions occur. Counselors can also discuss the expectation of clients and students to minimize distractions while receiving counseling services.

It is prudent to address the issue of dress, attire, and setting for videoconferencing sessions in relation to distractions. As in a F2F session, it goes without saying that counselors should be dressed appropriately for conducting a DC/TMH session. Consequently, a counselor may need to discuss dress, attire, and setting with their clients prior to beginning DC/TMH sessions. Some clients may elect to attend DC/TMH sessions while wearing pajamas, lounge attire, or less clothing than they would if they were to come to the office. When sessions are conducted in one's home, the client often dresses as they would in their own home. Similarly, clients might elect to lay in bed during session, get under the covers, eat lunch, or make coffee during session. In order to avoid these types of distractions, before engaging in DC/TMH sessions, the client and counselor should discuss expectations for attire, location, and activity during sessions. These discussions are based on client and counselor preference/comfort, as opposed to ethical codes or guidelines, but they are important discussions to have before an uncomfortable situation arises.

Verifying Identity

The American Counseling Association (ACA, 2014) and the National Board of Certified Counselors (NBCC, 2016) require counselors engaging in distance practice to verify client identity. At the start of each counseling session, counselors can verify the client identity by using the previously discussed protocols. For video conferencing sessions, counselors should ask the client to hold up a government issued photo ID for the first few sessions. The name and information should match the information on record for the client, and the photo should match the face of the person on the screen. For phone, text/chat, or email sessions, the client or student should designate a code word to be spoken or written at the beginning of each session. Sessions should not progress until the code word is provided.

Verify Privacy

It is the counselor's responsibility to both model confidentiality and privacy, and attempt to ensure confidentiality and privacy. For video conference sessions, counselors can scan their camera around the room to show the client that the work space is private and confidential, and that no third parties are able to overhear the session (Luxton et al., 2016). Similarly, counselors ask clients to scan their device around the room to ensure that their location is also private. For phone, email, or text/chat sessions, the counselor can simply state that they are working in a private setting, and ask the client if their location is also private. It is important to ask clients to turn off all smart-devices that might have voice-activated recording features, and for the counselor to ensure that their own voice-activated recording devices are disabled (Arcuri Sanders, 2020).

Verifying Location

The American Telemedicine Association (ATA, 2013) recommends discussing the risks with clients of changing locations, and how changes to the clients' location may impact safety and security measures. Client safety plans should include information on the nearest emergency facility, and changes to those locations impact the counselor's ability to provide support in an emergency. For this reason, counselors should verify location with clients at the beginning of each session to ensure that they have access to emergency personnel based on the client's location. This can be accomplished by simply asking the client where they are located at the time of the session.

Client/Counselor Relationship

Most counselors would agree that the foundation of any counseling process is the client–counselor relationship. The counselor's ability to demonstrate empathy, genuineness, and unconditional positive regard is essential to the counseling relationship. It has been demonstrated that a greater percentage of client change is generated by the relationship, as opposed to counseling skills and techniques (Ivey et al., 2018). A variety of counseling skills, such as empathy, attending, observation, reflecting feeling, and others, serve to enhance that client–counselor relationship. Ivey et al. (2018) state, "If you don't maintain the relationship, you will likely lose the client" (p. 230).

Earlier studies indicate that counselors believed DC/TMH may negatively impact the client–counselor relationship, and specifically that telephone, text, email, or video conference counseling significantly decreased a counselor's ability to build rapport (Centore & Milacci, 2008). More recent studies indicate that clients find DC/TMH contacts helpful (Gilat & Reshef, 2015), while others have found that clients have mixed responses to the DC/TMH relationship (Mishna et al., 2015). A focus on client-counselor relationship is critical to successful DC/TMH interactions. Trepal et al. (2007) recommend discussing clients' reactions and feelings about conducting sessions online early in the relationship as well as throughout the counseling process. They also recommend reviewing ethics and confidentiality statements and accepting digital signatures before beginning DC/TMH sessions.

It is possible to create a therapeutic alliance to enhance the client–counselor relationship while conducting DC/TMH sessions. For videoconference sessions, beyond ensuring a good quality image and video, counselors can confirm with clients that they can be seen and heard at each session, and ask about client comfort. Counselors can make nonverbal cues or attending words a bit more pronounced, and can also ask more questions that require reflection. Facial expressions and hand gestures can be used to portray empathy, as well as the client's ability to see the counselor's whole body language. It is also recommended that counselors spend time during session on rapport building and being aware of cultural variations (Simpson et al., 2016). Telephone sessions can also check in with client at the beginning of sessions to ensure audio connections are stable. It is recommended that using homework, particularly with cognitive behavioral interventions, can bridge the gap between telephone sessions (Saunders & Osborn, 2016). For email sessions, it is recommended that the counselor's thoughtfully reply to the individual communications of the client, as opposed to hasty or "canned" responses that may appear abrupt or insincere (Recupero & Harms, 2016). Derrig-Palumbo (2016) points out that relationships can flourish with written words, such as pen pal relationships. In order to foster relationships in written word such as email, chat, and texting, Derrig-Palumbo recommends using typed statements that express empathy, request permission, normalize, collaborate, search for strengths, and nurture hope (pp. 19–20).

These basic logistical components of establishing a professional workspace, avoiding distractions, verifying identity, privacy, location, and focusing on the client–counselor relationship are a necessary foundation for DC/TMH practice. Beyond the basics, the nuances of nonverbal communication and managing emotion may be challenged during DC/TMH. The counselor has a responsibility to address these challenges and develop adequate strategies to overcome them in order to maintain and enhance the client–counselor relationship.

NONVERBAL COMMUNICATION AND DISTANCE DEFICITS

One of the benefits of F2F counseling is the ability to fully see and hear the client. In most F2F sessions, the counselor can read the client's full body language in live time. The ability to both see the client and be seen by the client allows counselors to portray empathy and respond to their clients' emotional needs. Counselors observe clients' nonverbal behavior and verbal behavior, as well as conflict, discrepancy, and incongruence among this verbal and nonverbal communication (Ivey et al., 2018). DC/TMH may create barriers for the counselor in that the inability to see or hear the client significantly impacts the counselor's ability to observe verbal and nonverbal communication. Counselors must be aware of the potential barriers created by technology and make efforts to overcome them. The counselor can begin by being aware of their own image, body language, and nonverbal communication, as well as how these concepts are perceived in different modalities (e.g., phone, video, email, text).

Video Images

For video sessions, counselors and clients should be sitting a comfortable distance from the screen. Clients and counselors should be able to, at a minimum, see one another's full face and, ideally, see one another's body from the waist up. Images that are too close, too distant, or at an awkward angle exacerbate the barriers created by technology. Both parties must be able to comfortably hear one another based on their distance from the microphone. Wired headphones, as opposed to wireless headphones will impact the distance that client and counselor can comfortably move away from their screen. Devices should be placed on a firm surface that allows natural eye contact that is level with the video camera on the device (Simpson et al., 2016). Stands for tablets/phones or risers for laptops may help with stability and improving natural gaze toward the camera. Avoid placing devices on one's lap, soft surfaces (e.g., beds) where movement by a person will cause the image to shift or shake. Excessive camera movement is distracting for some viewers.

Eye Contact

Eye contact during videoconferencing may appear diverted. Because most counselors will look at the client on the screen, as opposed to the camera and the top of the device, it may appear as if the counselor is looking downward instead of making eye contact with the client. Counselors can overcome this obstacle by moving or dragging their client image to the top of their screen, directly below the camera. This helps to redirect the counselor's natural gaze toward the top of the screen where the camera is located. Eye contact is absent in phone sessions. In phone sessions, it is important to use a balance of attending words, encouragers, and paraphrasing (Ivey et al., 2018), such that the client knows the counselor is listening and focusing on their words. Any of these skills can be overdone (Ivey et al., 2018), thus counselors need to find a balance in using these skills, and avoid unintentionally interrupting a client with their use.

Nonverbal Communication

Beyond eye contact, nonverbal communication includes body language, facial expressions, and the tone/pitch/pace of language. These nonverbal components are an important part to the client/counselor relationship and help the counselor understand the client's emotion during a F2F session (Ivey et al., 2018). For email, text, and chat sessions, nonverbal communication is absent, although some may argue that use of emoticons, emoji's, and certain typefaces can provide insight into client emotion. Counselors may wish to encourage those tools during email/text/chat sessions for clients who use them. For telephone sessions, counselors pay close attention to vocal cues that signify emotion or struggle. Those vocal cues include the intensity, rate, tone, pace, and pitch of one's verbal communication. Even during video sessions, a counselor may be unable to see a client's entire body and unable to notice subtle movements, such as shifting in one's seat, wringing hands, clenched fists, or fidgeting legs and feet. Depending on the quality of the video connection, the counselor may be unable to detect small nonverbal cues, such as watering eyes or deep sighs.

These challenges in nonverbal communication and the barriers of technology should be addressed with clients in their informed consent document, early in counseling and as regular reminders throughout treatment. The counselor's ability to honestly discuss the challenges of technology with the client invites the client to be an equal partner in the counseling relationship and work collaboratively with the counselor to overcome these shortfalls. In addition, counselors can use strategies to identify emotion, and create connections with clients that foster genuine relationships.

IDENTIFYING EMOTION

The absence or reduction of nonverbal communication in DC/TMH settings requires the counselor to have a keen awareness of the client's feelings and emotions. Because nonverbal cues are lost, counselors need to probe more effectively for emotion during DC/TMH sessions. This requires variations beyond the basic "How do you feel about that?" probe. Counselors must have a robust feelings-word vocabulary in order to effectively reflect feeling with their clients (Ivey et al., 2018). Counselors can consider building regular feeling-checks in to their DC/TMH sessions, e.g., at the beginning, middle, and end. Clients will come to expect these emotional probes throughout session and may be more connected to their emotional responses as a result. Counselors can also model expressing emotion and feeling for clients in the DC/TMH setting (Trepal et al., 2007), by using a rich feeling-word vocabulary and appropriately self-disclosing their own feelings in relation to counseling content.

Counselors need to be creative in order to tap into both verbal and nonverbal emotion. As stated, being honest with the client about the DC/TMH nonverbal communication challenge involves them in the solution. For example, during a telephone session, a counselor might offer the following:

> What you've described sounds very painful, and I'm noticing that you've been quiet since sharing it. Because I can't see you during this telephone session, I wonder if you'd be able to tell me how your body language is right now and what I would see if you were sitting across from me? How is your body language connected to what you are feeling at this moment?

Similarly, during an email session, a counselor might type, "In your last message you told me you were angry. Can you tell me where that anger sits in your body? If I was sitting across from you right now, instead of at the keyboard, how would I see your anger on your body?" These questions challenge the client to connect to their emotion within their body. If clients regularly practice sharing their emotion and their body language, they may offer this information in future sessions as a way to connect to the counselor, share what they are feeling, and enhance the client–counselor relationship.

Counselors need to be familiar with the most recent text language and communication if conducting sessions via text or chat (Trepal et al., 2007). A variety of abbreviations, emoji's, and emoticons portray emotion in place of words (Provine et al., 2007). Counselors must not only understand that language but must utilize a technological device that can receive those symbols. While most devices (e.g., Apple, Android) can communicate across platforms (e.g., PC, Mac), there may still be subtle differences or difficulties in deciphering symbols and messages (Nield, 2018). These patterns quickly change and it benefits the counselor to attempt to stay on top of these communication patterns if they are working with a population that may regularly use them (e.g., adolescents; Cornell University, 2019).

Visual aids may be helpful in assisting clients or students in identifying feelings. In F2F sessions, counselors often display visual images or motivational statements in their office and waiting area. Counselors can use visual cues to assist clients in identifying emotions such as the feelings wheel (Wilcox, 1982), emotion face charts, or emotion word lists. These tools help clients connect with their emotions and expand their feelings vocabulary. These visual aids can be utilized in a DC/TMH setting but may require email or share screen settings. Counselors can reference these visual aids during feeling checks, or when asking clients to identify with feelings they are experiencing.

Silence and Timing

The use of silence can be therapeutic in the counseling relationship. During F2F sessions, counselors intentionally use silence to allow for reflection, emotion, or processing (Ivey et al., 2018). During those F2F sessions, counselors observe how clients respond to silence, by observing their body language and eye contact. Silence during DC/TMH sessions can be nerve wracking and anxiety producing for both the client and the counselor, particularly for sessions lacking visual cues. During a telephone session, the client or counselor may misinterpret silence as the other being disconnected or disengaged from the session. During video sessions, either party may wonder if the video image is frozen, lagging, or disconnected.

Counselors can discuss the challenge of silence in DC/TMH in their informed consent and throughout sessions. A counselor who is intentionally using silence during a video session may seek to make small movements (e.g., casually moving hand up to chin, cheek or mouth, shifting in their seat slightly). These small movements cue the client that the counselor is indeed there, in live time, and that the computer connection is functional. For telephone sessions, counselors can use small encouragers (e.g., mm-hmm, I see, take your time) to probe silent spaces and cue the client that you are present and engaged. They may even introduce or invite the silence during a phone session by saying "Let's just take a few moments to silently reflect on that." During written sessions, such as text, messaging and email, the informed consent documents should specify time frames for responding to messages such that clients know when they can reasonably expect counselor responses.

Silence may unintentionally invite interruptions. Because there is often a slight delay in the sending and receiving of a message over technology, it is likely that one party may start speaking and/or typing before another party has finished. For this reason, it is wise to pause and allow for slight silence before responding to client statements. Messages may also be delayed by slower technology and Internet speed. If connections are slow and messages are delayed, counselors need to allow more silence after each communication. With text and messaging, use of an ellipse (. . .) at the end of a typed message often indicates that the person is planning on continuing. Clients and counselors can develop systems for typed and spoken communication. For example, some communication systems utilize "done" or "GA" ("go ahead") at the end of one's statement. These protocols have been in place for TTY (teletypewriter) communication for several years (National Business & Disability Council, 2014), as well as online support groups.

The length of DC/TMH sessions may vary. For email or text sessions, the amount of time it takes to type a response is generally longer than the time it takes for someone to respond verbally. Based on the need to focus on issues such as eye contact, nonverbal communication, identifying emotion, and silence, DC/TMH sessions can require counselors to move at a slower pace. Counselors want to avoid bombarding clients with questions, and only asking a few questions at a time in email/chat/asynchronous formats, as well as allow ample time to close the session (Trepal et al., 2007).

CHALLENGES AND OPPORTUNITIES

The counseling profession quickly adapted to delivering DC/TMH services in a post-COVID-19 era. There is no doubt that DC/TMH delivery has improved client access to individual counseling. Yet there is also little doubt that technology can be problematic, as has been seen with the emergence of behaviors such as cyberbullying, cyber stalking, and "catfishing" relationships (the act of posing as someone online; Anthony, 2015). Some of the challenges of DC/TMH have been addressed earlier in this chapter, such as nonverbal communication and identifying emotion. While there are other perceived challenges to offering individual DC/TMH counseling, there are also opportunities for DC/TMH to improve individual counseling.

Technological Connections

The importance of using secure, reliable technology to communicate with clients via DC/TMH has been previously addressed. However, the reality is that lost connections and communication delays will likely occur. When they do, it is important that the counselor and client have a predetermined plan for reconnection (Reamer, 2018). This plan may be outlined in an informed consent document, and can be reinforced sporadically, such as at the beginning of each session or as technical issues begin to arise (e.g., freezing or delayed images/communication). Such plans include who initiates contact after disconnection, and what modality will be used to reconnect (e.g., video, phone, text). Elliot, Abbass, and Rousmaniere offer the following suggestions to maximize internet connections:

> Using computer with adequate processing capacity. Turn off other computer programs. Turn off other computers if on a network. Use broadband Internet. Use cloud sharing to send video rather than screen share. Use cable versus wireless Internet connection. Schedule web conferences outside of peak Internet usage times. (2018, p. 176)

Feedback and Background Noise

Feedback is another challenge that may arise on individual TMH sessions, specifically if using videoconferencing. Feedback usually occurs when the sound coming out of a device's speaker is also picked up by its microphone. Feedback may sound like an echo or a high-pitched noise. Feedback is best addressed by having one or both parties turn down their microphone volume, turn down their speaker volume, speak softer, or put themselves on mute. Background noise is simply noise occurring in the background that is distracting to the call or session. Because some technologies are designed to focus on the person speaking, background noises will get picked up on video calls, conference calls, and phone calls. The technology mistakes this background noise for "talking" and blocks out others' microphones to focus on the person speaking. Reducing background noise is best accomplished by moving to a quiet location or putting oneself on mute. Obviously, one party on mute may inhibit verbal communication during individual counseling sessions, which reinforces the need for private and confidential workspaces.

Clients in Crisis

The idea of helping a client in crisis, while being physically separated from that client, concerns many DC/TMH counselors. Adequate preparation and safety planning for all clients, not just those in crisis, is essential to establishing an ethical, safe, and effective practice (Turvey, 2018). Yet helping clients in crisis from a distance is not a new concept. Crisis phone lines and more recently crisis text lines serve thousands of clients in crisis each year remotely (Hornblow, 1986; Predmore et al., 2017). While the individual counselor may not have access to the same technology and emergency deployment systems as these national hotlines, they possess many of the counseling skills used by crisis line workers (e.g., empathy, attending, compassion), as well as one tool that these hotlines don't have: the client–counselor relationship. Counselors who develop effective relationships with their clients via DC/TMH counseling have an opportunity to portray empathy and caring in a meaningful way to clients. While not a protection against harm to self or others, the client–counselor relationship has been cited as being one of the most impactful in client treatment (Ivey et al., 2018). Counselors will use their relationship with their client, as well as the formerly developed safety plans, protocols and emergency resources, to assist clients in crisis.

Individualizing Services

The challenges of navigating technology, encryption, and detailed informed consents can overwhelm the counselor considering DC/TMH. Yet the benefits of individualized services with DC/TMH are vast. Through DC/TMH, counselors have an opportunity to reach clients without other access to counseling. DC/TMH provides the flexibility to alter traditional F2F formats to meet the needs of the individual. The counseling profession advocates for individualized, holistic, and humanistic approaches to our counseling practice. The Association for Spiritual, Ethical, and Religious Values in Counseling (ASERVIC)'s white paper on spiritualty states

> majority of persons in America profess some form of religious belief, even if they are not active participants in a particular religion. . . . Their beliefs have a profound impact on their world view, relationships, self-concept, and problem solving approaches. (ASERVIC, n.d., para. 8)

Similarly, the Association for Humanistic Counseling (AHC) emphasizes the value and dignity of the individual, as well as the individual's responsibility and autonomy to create their own outcomes in life. DC/TMH allows us to include the client's world view and self-concept as they create their own destiny and improve their own lives. Technology creates opportunities to both individualize and enhance services.

Enhancing Services

The use of technology as the modality for our counseling sessions is exciting. Many prospective DC/TMH counselors consider the myriad of clients that they might serve due to the expansive reach of DC/TMH practice. However, technology allows the counselor opportunities to enhance their individual sessions in ways that F2F sessions less easily provide. For example, most videoconferencing software allows users to "share screen" which enables the opposite party to see the screen of the "sharer." Through this feature, clients and counselors can share information and resources in ways not previously achieved. Clients can take an online screening tool in the presence of a counselor that is scored immediately. Counselors can walk clients through the use of an online resource. Email allows counselors to provide links to valuable resources. Clients can use their creativity to express feelings or share content during sessions, including music, videos, photos, or writing (Kozolowski & Homes, 2017). Technology provides countless opportunities to expand beyond our traditional F2F skills, creating personalized, individualized and enhanced sessions for our clients.

Documentation

The use of DC/TMH does not eliminate the counselor's responsibility for documentation. The counselor continues to be responsible for creating secure documentation and storing/sending secure information. However, the use of technology may facilitate documentation storage and retrieval, such as sending and reviewing an email with an informed consent document. Sending this information in advance allows the client and counselor to spend time on questions on the document and gives the client an opportunity to read through the document at their own pace (Trepal et al., 2007).

CASE STUDY: INDIVIDUAL COUNSELING

Counselor A has transitioned one of their clients, Client B, to telephone counseling as a result of the COVID-19 pandemic. Counselor A has not previously had training or experience in distance counseling or telemental health, but they did receive training on developing a detailed Informed Consent document for DC/TMH, including a safety plan. Counselor A reviewed the Informed Consent and developed a safety plan with Client B before starting telephone sessions. Counselor A had only been seeing Client B for 2 weeks before the transition to DC/TMH. During their first two F2F sessions, Client B was reserved and guarded, although they cooperated with the intake process. Client B stated that they had come to counseling to be a better parent to their children and better partner to their spouse. There was no evidence or history of mental illness, substance use, abuse, suicidal or homicidal ideation for Client B or their family during the intake. Client B was hesitant to use DC/TMH, but agreed to try phone sessions, in order to "keep things moving."

During their first telephone session, Counselor A attempted to enhance rapport by asking Client B about their coping in relation to COVID-19. Client B provided only short, one-word answers in response to the counselor's probes. Counselor A attempted to move on to Client B's presenting problem of parenting and partnering. Whenever Counselor A would ask Client B for more information or to elaborate, Client B would simply respond, "I don't know" or "I couldn't say." Client B was often silent for long periods of time, leaving Counselor A to wonder if they were still on the call. Counselor A utilized their counseling skills to engage Client B but continued to receive short, guarded responses, or no response at all.

Counselor A thought that Client B sounded frustrated but did not attempt to confirm their emotions for fear that Client B would want to discontinue DC/TMH sessions. As a result, Counselor A suggested ending the session early and trying again next week. Client B agreed.

During their second telephone session, Client B was more communicative. Client B provided more information in response to Counselor A's open-ended questions, and shared more about the challenges they were having with the partner. Client B also shared a desire to protect their children from knowing that there was discord between the parents. Counselor A noted background noises during the session, including a humming sound and soft music. When Counselor A asked about these noises, Client B explained that they were driving around in their car during the session because that is the only private place they had to speak. Client B explained that during their last session, their children were in their bedroom on the computer and their partner was in the next room watching TV, so they were not able to speak openly. Client B stated "That's why I kept telling you 'I couldn't say' because I really couldn't say with my partner in the next room."

DISCUSSION QUESTIONS

1. What do you think about the counselor's decision to transition to DC/TMH during the COVID-19 pandemic? What factors would they need to consider before making that transition?

2. Think about the counselor's preparation for the DC/TMH session. How well did they prepare? How do you think the client felt about the transition to DC/TMH?

3. Counselor A struggled during the first phone session. What steps could the counselor have taken to avoid those struggles or improve that session?

4. Client B spoke more comfortably during the second phone session, but also shared that they were driving around in their car. What concerns does that pose for the counselor? How would you respond as the counselor when you learned why they were in the car?

5. Assuming good intent, what did Counselor A do well?

CRITICAL QUESTIONS IN DECIDING TO PRACTICE

This chapter discussed beginning individual counseling via DC/TMH. The chapter provided an overview of the logistics of the practice, as well as the fundamentals of conducting a DC/TMH session. Anthony (2015) encourages counselors to ask themselves, "'My client is online—am I online in a sufficient capacity to treat him or her effectively?'" (Anthony, 2015, p. 40). As you consider your own transition to DC/TMH with your individual clients, consider the following:

1. How can you make your DC/TMH workspace professional and confidential? What changes do you need to make to your workspace for videoconferencing sessions as opposed to phone or email/text sessions?

2. What distractions might occur in your DC/TMH workspace? What steps do you have to take to reduce distractions, while also reducing the likelihood of disconnections, poor connections and feedback?

3. What is your plan to verify identity, location, and privacy with your clients each time you connect with them in DC/TMH sessions?

4. What skills and techniques will you use to enhance the client–counselor relationship? How will you attempt to display unconditional positive regard through DC/TMH sessions?

5. How will you help clients connect with their emotion during DC/TMH sessions? What special skills and strategies will you use to reflect feeling and demonstrate empathy? How will those skills vary by modality (e.g., video conference, phone, email, text)?

6. How will you incorporate silence into DC/TMH sessions? How will you address the concept of silence during DC/TMH sessions with clients? Will you address it before it occurs, in the moment, or after?

7. What is the ideal location in your home for WiFi and mobile connections? Do you have access to a wired phone or Internet, if needed?

8. What is your plan for managing clients in crisis? How will you get them remote support in the event of their intent to harm themselves or others?

9. Brainstorm ways to individualize your counseling sessions. How can you use your DC/TMH sessions to better understand your client's world views, relationships, and problem-solving abilities? How can you use these sessions to foster their dignity and improve their overall quality of life?

10. How can you use technology to enhance your DC/TMH sessions? What are some strategies that you can use to improve the service you would give to a client/student during a DC/TMH as opposed to a F2F session?

VOICES FROM THE FIELD

Trauma Work and Individual Counseling

Michaia Walker, LCSW

I have been working as a psychotherapist on the teletherapy platform since 2018. I believe trauma work is central to any lens through which you approach therapy. Clients are sometimes aware of this and can identify trauma as one of the reasons they are seeking support. Other clients are unaware until the trauma or triggers present themselves in session, which can encourage further work or stop the process entirely for someone who feels unprepared or overwhelmed. Often the trauma is childhood abuse (physical, sexual, psychological) of some kind and/or intimate partner violence.

I've worked with all types of trauma survivors both in person and via teletherapy. I think one of the biggest challenges via teletherapy is when the client only wants to work via messaging. It's often not effective or consistent and clients quickly disengage from the process. It's easier to disengage when the only way your therapist can freely contact you is via email notifications. Some clients, more frequently in the last year or so, are willing to do the work via phone. This is obviously a more successful type of connection and requires much more effort on the part of the client to make the appointment and show up on time. Clients can only be contacted via the platform/app, so if they do not make the effort to login/show up, there is no live session that day. This is on par with clients who choose to do video sessions as well. With all mental health treatment milieus and modalities, the onus is on the client to make at least a little effort toward their growth.

One positive about addressing trauma with clients online is that they access their treatment from a safe and comfortable place. Often clients chose to have sessions while they are home, but others choose to have sessions in parks, while they are walking, while they are with their pet, and so forth. I believe the natural environment allows for a deeper exploration of the trauma and healing for the client who is committed to the work. This can also increase the process for rapport building.

With the recent shift to solely teletherapy amid this COVID-19 pandemic, clients are having to rely on these online platforms or switch to online sessions with their therapists. This has created a real revolution in the mental health community. All kinds of treatment are now only accessible via telehealth. This shift to mandatory teletherapy has also increased the level of fidelity and commitment of some clients. A shared traumatic event worldwide is bringing more people to seek mental health treatment with the awareness that they are seeking support for their trauma.

CONCLUSION

Individual counseling occurs in many counseling settings including mental health, school, college, and others. The use of DC and TMH for individual counseling requires that the counselor manage the logistics of the DC/TMH relationship. This includes identifying a professional workspace, avoiding distractions, and verifying client identity, privacy, and location. The counselor must also focus on the client–counselor relationship, and make efforts toward enhancing and maintaining the relationship via technological interactions. Technology can pose challenges to communication during counseling relationships, and the counselor must ensure that the video image, eye contact, and nonverbal communication are adapted to meet these challenges. Technology may also create limits on the counselor's ability to identify emotion and effectively utilize silence, and the counselor can address these limitations by probing for emotion, using visual aids, and addressing silence. Challenges such as technological concerns and background noise may arise, as well as more serious concerns, such as a client in crisis. Counselors address these concerns with technology tips, as well as utilizing thorough informed consent documents that include a safety plan. Counselors can utilize DC/TMH to both enhance and personalize their individual counseling sessions, but must also follow protocols for appropriate documentation.

REFERENCES

Arcuri Sanders, N. M. (2020, January 14). Hey Siri: Did you break confidentiality or did I? *Counseling Today.* https://ct.counseling.org/2020/01/hey-siri -did-you-break-confidentiality-or-did-i

American Counseling Association. (2014). *2014 ACA code of ethics.* https://www .counseling.org/Resources/aca-code-of-ethics.pdf

American Telemedicine Association. (2013, May). *Practice guidelines for video based online mental health services.* https://www.integration.samhsa.gov/operations -administration/practice-guidelines-for-video-based-online-mental-health -services_ata_5_29_13.pdf

Anthony, K. (2015). Training therapists to work effectively online and offline within digital culture. *British Journal of Guidance & Counselling, 43*(1), 36–42, https:// doi.org/10.1080/03069885.2014.924617

Association for Spiritual, Ethical, and Religious Values in Counseling. (n.d.). *A white paper of the Association for Spiritual, Ethical, and Religious Values in Counseling.* http://www.aservic.org/wp-content/uploads/2015/02/ASERVIC- WHITE-PAPER.pdf

Baird, M. B., Whitney, L., & Caedo, C. E. (2018). Experiences and attitudes among psychiatric mental health advanced practice nurses in the use of telemental health: Results of an online survey. *Journal of the American Psychiatric Nurses Association, 24*(3), 235–240. https://doi.org/10.1177/1078390317717330

Centore, A. J., & Milacci, A. (2008). A study of mental health counselor's use and perspectives on distance counseling. *Journal of Mental Health Counseling, 30,* 267–282. https://doi.org/10.17744/mehc.30.3.q871r684n863u75r

Cornell University. (2019). *New York State Consortium for Advancing and Supported Employment: Creating a framework of services for students and youth.* L. Lisa Yang and Hock E. Tan Institute on Employment and Disability.

Council on the Accreditation of Counseling and Related Education Programs. (2020, March). *Updates on COVID-19: Professional practice standards advisory.* https://www.cacrep.org/for-programs/updates-on-covid-19/#march63

Derrig-Palumbo, K. (2016). Using chat and instant messaging (IM) to conduct a therapeutic relationship. In S. Goss, K. Anthony, L. Sykes Stretch, & D. Merz Nagel (Eds.), *Technology in mental health: Applications in practice supervision and training* (2nd ed.). Charles C. Thomas Publisher, LTD.

Elliot, J., Abbass, A., & Rousmaniere, T. (2018). Technology assisted deliberate practice for improving psychotherapy effectiveness. In J. J. Magnavita (Ed.), *Using technology in mental health practice.* American Psychological Association.

Gilat, I., & Reshef, E. (2015). The perceived helpfulness of rendering emotional first aid via email. *British Journal of Guidance & Counselling, 43,* 94–104. https://doi.org/10.1080/03069885.2014.909006

Hornblow, A. R. (1986). The evolution and effectiveness of telephone counseling services. *Hospital and Community Psychiatry, 37,* 731–733. https://doi.org/10.1176/ps.37.7.731

Ivey, A. E., Ivey, M. B., & Zalaquett, C. P. (2018). *Intentional interviewing and counseling: Facilitating client development in a multicultural society* (9th ed.). Brooks/Cole.

Kozolowski, K. A., & Homes, C. M. (2014). Experiences in online process groups: A qualitative study. *Journal for Specialists in Group Work, 39,* 276–300. https://doi.org/10.1080/01933922.2014.948235

Kozolowski, K. A., & Homes, C. M. (2017). Teaching online group counseling skills in an on campus group counseling course. *The Journal of Counseling preparation and Supervision, 9*(1). http://dx.doi.org/10.7729/911.1157

Luxton, D. D., Nelson, E. L., & Maheu, M. M. (2016). *A practitioner's guide to telemental health: How to conduct legal, ethical, and evidence-based telepractice.* American Psychological Association.

Mishna, F., Bogo, M., & Sawyer, J. (2015). Cyber counseling: Illuminating benefits and challenges. *Clinical Social Work Journal, 43,* 169–178. https://doi.org/10.1007/s10615-013-0470-1

National Board of Certified Counselors. (2016). *Policy regarding the provision of distance professional services.* https://www.nbcc.org/Assets/Ethics/NBCCPolicyRegardingPracticeofDistanceCounselingBoard.pdf

National Business & Disability Council at the Viscardi Center. (2014). *Etiquette tips when using a TTY.* https://www.viscardicenter.org/wp-content/uploads/2016/09/2014_NBDC_Flyer_Etiquette_Tips_TTY-1.pdf

Nield, D. (2018, March 22). Make your Android and iOS devices work together. *Popular Science.* https://www.popsci.com/make-android-ios-work-together

Perle, J. G., Langsam, L. C., Randel, A., Lutchman, S., Levine, A B., Odland, A. P., Nierenberg, B., & Marker, C. D. (2012). Attitudes toward psychological telehealth: Current and future clinical psychologists opinions of internet-based interventions. *Journal of Clinical Psychology, 69,* 100–113. https://doi.org/10.1002/jclp.21912

Predmore, Z., Ramchand, R., Ayer, L., Kotzias, V., Engel, C., Ebener, P., Kemp, J. E., Karras, E., & Haas, G. L. (2017). Expanding suicide crisis services to text and chat. *Crisis, 38*(4), 255–260. https://doi.org/10.1027/0227-5910/a000460

Provine, R. R., Spencer, R. J., & Mandell, D. L. (2007). Emotional expression online: Emoticons punctuate website text messages. *Journal of Language and Social Psychology, 26,* 299–307. https://doi.org/10.1177/0261927X06303481

Reamer, F. G. (2018). Evolving standards of care in the age of cybertechnology. *Behavioral Science Law, 36,* 257–269. https://doi.org/10.1002/bsl.2336

Recupero, P. R., & Harms, S. (2016). Using email to conduct a therapeutic relationship. In S. Goss, K. Anthony, L. Sykes Stretch, & D. Merz Nagel (Eds.), *Technology in mental health: Applications in practice supervision and training* (2nd ed.). Charles C. Thomas Publisher, LTD.

Saunders, D. E., & Osborn, D. S. (2016). Using the telephone for conducting a therapeutic relationship. In S. Goss, K. Anthony, L. Sykes Stretch, & D. Merz Nagel (Eds.), *Technology in mental health: Applications in practice supervision and training* (2nd Ed.). Charles C. Thomas Publisher, LTD.

Simms, D. C., Gibson, K., & O'Donnell, S. (2011). To use or not to use: Clinicians' perceptions of telemental health. *Canadian Psychology, 52,* 41–51. https://doi.org/10.1037/a0022275

Simpson, S., Richardson, L., & Reid, C. (2016). Therapeutic alliance in videoconferencing based psychotherapy. In S. Goss, K. Anthony, L. Sykes Stretch, & D. Merz Nagel (Eds.), *Technology in mental health: Applications in practice supervision and training* (2nd ed.). Charles C. Thomas Publisher, LTD.

Trepal, H., Haberstroh, S., Duffey, T., & Evans, M. (2007). Considerations and strategies for teaching online counseling skills: Establishing relationships in cyberspace. *Counselor Education & Supervision, 46,* 266–279. https://doi.org/10.1002/j.1556-6978.2007.tb00031.x

Turvey, C. L. (2018). Telemental health care delivery: Evidence base and practical considerations. In J. J. Magnavita (Ed.), *Using technology in mental health practice.* American Psychological Association.

U.S. Department of Health and Human Services, Office of Civil Rights. (2020, March 17). *Notification of enforcement discretion for telehealth remote communication during the COVID-19 nationwide public health emergency.* https://www.hhs.gov/hipaa/for-professionals/special-topics/emergency-preparedness/notification-enforcement-discretion-telehealth/index.html

Wilcox, G. (1982). The feelings wheel: A tool for expanding awareness of emotions and increasing spontaneity and intimacy. *Transactional Analysis Journal, 12*(4), 274–286. https://doi.org/10.1177/036215378201200411

6

Group Counseling via Telemental Health

INTRODUCTION

Counselors from all specialties utilize group counseling with clients and students. Most counselors, whether employed in mental health, substance use, school, rehabilitation, college, or other specializations, will utilize group counseling with the clients and students they serve. Group counseling can be utilized with participants ranging from young children to older adults, and can be effective for issues from social skills to job searching to complex mental health conditions. The benefits of group counseling are vast, including shared learning experiences for students/clients and reduced costs for agencies/clinicians. Group counseling is also considered efficient, as group members benefit from the insights of the counselor as well as other group members. Group counseling can be brief, time-limited and focused on a specific goal shared by members. Groups allow individuals who struggle with relationships the benefit of interacting with others and learning from behaviors or communication patterns that other members model (Corey et al., 2010).

The benefits of group are perhaps best articulated via Yalom's (1995) therapeutic factors. Yalom posits that group therapy facilitates eleven therapeutic factors, including installation of hope, universality, imparting of information, altruism, corrective recapitulation of the primary family group, development of socializing techniques, imitative behavior, interpersonal learning, group cohesiveness, catharsis, and existential factors (p. 1). These therapeutic factors demonstrate the shared experiences that clients and students can gain from the group experience, particularly for those who are committed to the process and feel a sense of belonging in the group. Many individual counselors made the transition to distance counseling (DC) and telemental health (TMH) during the March 2020 COVID-19 shelter-in-place orders. Group counselors also transitioned to DC/TMH during this time, however group counseling via distance modalities were operating long before the COVID-19 crisis.

Alcoholics Anonymous (AA) reported its first ham radio group in 1967; in addition, electronic bulletin boards created instant meetings for AA members around the globe beginning in the mid-1980s (AA, 2020). Telephone meetings, videoconference meetings, and synchronous and asynchronous discussion boards are common among self-help groups such as AA, Overeaters Anonymous (OA), Narcotics Anonymous (NA), and Heroin Anonymous (HA). Online support groups have been serving individuals since the mid-1990s, beginning with email listserves and advancing to web-based platforms (Boniel-Nissim, 2016). One of the largest online support recovery networks, In the Rooms, was founded in October of 2008, and reports having over 650,000 members worldwide that attend their AA, NA, OA, Gamblers Anonymous (GA), Sex Addicts Anonymous, and Medically Assisted Recovery Anonymous sessions (In the Rooms, 2020). Online support groups exist for issues beyond addictions, such as emotional concerns, medical difficulties, coping strategies, and family members of those with specific conditions (Boniel-Nissim, 2016). While the focus of this chapter is on DC/TMH groups, support groups have a long history of online and distance practice, which provides valuable insight into the discussion of distance group counseling.

DISTANCE GROUPS

Traditional face-to-face (F2F) group counseling requires screening members for group appropriateness, as well as reviewing an informed consent document with the clients, students, and/or guardians. These guidelines are also required for professional counselors conducting DC/TMH groups. Per the American Counseling Association's (ACA) Code of Ethics, professional counselors are responsible for including the risks and benefits of DC in the informed consent. Counselors ensure that the client or student has the technical, developmental, and cognitive ability to use the technology, as well as access to the required technology. Counselors themselves must be trained in both the technology and the capacity to facilitate groups via DC (ACA, 2014).

Types of Groups

It is important to recognize the distinction between DC/TMH groups and support groups. Support groups are mutual support groups that are not necessarily facilitated by a trained professional, and may be open to anyone with no prescreening (Boniel-Nissim, 2016). Often, support groups have no designated leader, leadership varies, or leaders emerge from the group itself. In other settings, leaders are individuals who have previously, or currently, been in need of the same support as the group members. While support groups may not be facilitated by professional counselors, many organizations have published standards and guidelines that benefit the counselor who is new to facilitating DC/TMH groups.

Groups can be classified as task/working groups, psychoeducation groups, counseling groups, psychotherapy groups, or mixed groups (Gladding, 2012). Task or working groups complete tasks or job assignments, and may also be called teams. Psychoeducation groups were originally designed for school settings and are also called educational groups or guidance groups (Gladding, 2012). Counseling groups are "preventive, growth oriented, and remedial" (Gladding, 2012, p. 14). Counseling groups may focus on learning a cognitive, affective, or behavioral skill, and also may focus on interpersonal processes, including shared difficulties in issues such as living, career, education, and relationships (Kozlowski & Homes, 2014). Psychotherapy groups, or group therapy, assist people with shared psychological concerns, often located in mental health facilities or hospitals (Gladding, 2012). Psychotherapy groups view the group cohesion and belongingness as part of the therapeutic process (Yalom, 1995) and address the psychopathology that is impacting one's life functioning (Kozlowski & Homes, 2014). Mixed groups don't necessarily fit into one format and may change their focus based on the members enrolled and their needs (Gladding, 2012).

Group Dynamics

The presence of others contributes to the healing process through elements such as universality (shared experiences), altruism (helping others), imitative behavior (modeling), or interpersonal learning (learning from one another), as indicated via Yalom's therapeutic factors (1995). Group dynamics, defined as "forces within the group" (Gladding, 2012, p. 29), are comprised of group content and group process. Group content involves the information that is shared and exchanged during the group time. Group content includes the content shared by the facilitator, as well as by the group members. Group process includes how the members interact with one another, including how the members anticipate and/or react to one another's needs. As groups evolve, the focus often shifts from the content of the group, to the process of the group, with an emphasis on the intergroup relationships, as well as intrapersonal learning. A critical component of group dynamics is creating trust between each member and the facilitator, as well as among members themselves (Corey et al., 2010). In order for people to fully participate in the group process, they need to trust that they are able to speak freely and without judgment.

Trust is essential to groups moving through stages of group development, often referred to as norming, storming, and performing, as well as termination (Gladding, 2012). All groups experience developmental phases as members move into their preferred roles within the group. During the forming phase, also known as orientation, members are new, trust is low, and uncertainty is high. Members are learning the group format and rules, and are likely on their best behavior. During the storming phase, tensions may increase or conflicts may occur as members assume different roles within the group. Members are deciding where they belong in the group and how they wish to invest in the group process. Conflicts may arise around issues of power and control, and issues such as monopolizing, dependency, and attacks on others arise. During the working phase, the group is usually most effective. Members have found a rhythm to the group dynamics, trust is higher, and the group is effectively working on their challenges and goals. Groups will also begin to prepare for termination.

The counselor who is facilitating a DC/TMH group needs to consider the type and purpose of the group. Psychoeducation groups may require mechanisms for participants to view materials, including visual aids, documents, or videos. As such, a counselor leading a psychoeducation DC/TMH group selects technology that supports those needs. This may include video technology with shared screen features or an internal messaging system that allows posted documents. Psychotherapy groups may benefit from being able to both see and hear all members of the group simultaneously, and the counselor may wish to explore technology that allows for diverse viewing options. To support the group process and shared learning, a counselor can utilize electronic journaling (Haberstroh et al., 2006) or digital discussion boards to foster intergroup dialogue. The facilitator also needs to consider whether the selected technology can be used to monitor group dynamics and foster trust among members.

Modalities for Distance Counseling/Telemental Health Groups

Distance counseling and telemental health groups use a variety of modalities including videoconferencing, telephone, chatrooms, and synchronous or asynchronous discussion boards. Videoconference groups are facilitated via secure videoconferencing technologies, where individuals enter the group via invitation or software platforms. In the wake of COVID-19, free videoconferencing software was widely used for group meetings and discussions, yet the security and privacy of some systems were lacking. Telephone groups regularly utilize conference-style phone systems, where individuals are provided with a phone number and access number, and then join a facilitated conference call.

Discussion boards are used for DC/TMH groups, but not regularly used with DC/TMH individual counseling. Discussion boards can be both synchronous and asynchronous (Boniel-Nissim, 2016). Synchronous discussion boards resemble "chat rooms," in which participants and facilitators sign on and type their comments in live time. Synchronous discussion boards are open for a specific time and duration, with a designated ending time. Asynchronous discussion boards allow users and facilitators to sign on based on their own needs and schedules; these boards may stay open indefinitely or may be closed by a moderator and facilitator after a designated period of time. In contrast to text or email messages, discussion boards utilize a shared location or "board" which is located on a designated platform. Users often need to sign in to that platform to access the discussion board, although some discussion boards are public. Some discussion boards display items with the most recent posts at the top, and older responses at the bottom (Boniel-Nissim, 2016).

Text or email messages are sent via the Internet to a group of recipients who utilize multiple platforms. Email, chat, or text is used with individual DC/TMH counseling. While these modalities may be used with DC/TMH groups, there is limited research to support its utility for group counseling purposes.

OPEN AND CLOSED GROUPS ONLINE

All groups, including online and F2F, have the option of being open or closed. When searching for support groups, such as AA, NA, OA, and others, groups are coded as open or closed groups. An open group is a group that is open to the public. Individuals are able to come and go from an open group, and may start or stop their group attendance at any time (Gladding, 2012). Closed groups are designated for specific members, either members of a specified group or members who have been screened for appropriateness. Closed group vary in format; some closed groups have a specific start and end period, and no new members can join during that time. Other closed groups have rolling entry and exit points, whereas individuals enter and exit at various times, but the group is closed to outside members (Gladding, 2012).

The concept of open and closed groups can create challenges in an online group counseling setting. Many, although not all, self-help groups are open groups, meaning that members do not require prescreening and may enter and exit as they please. Open group discussion boards present challenges for confidentiality. Incoming members may be unfamiliar with group rules and protocols. Additionally, they may engage in practices that interrupt the group dynamics or pose confidentiality concerns, such as recordings and screenshots of digital images. Similar to F2F sessions, open groups create issues with confidentiality and learned content. When people enter and exit the group at will, the group dynamics, cohesion, and process are interrupted. While there is no guarantee of confidentiality in any group setting (Corey et al., 2013), whether online or F2F, the entry and exit of individuals in online groups may exacerbate fears of confidentiality and impact trust. Participants have expressed feeling less connected to group members during online group experiences, and also that the group was superficial (Kozlowski & Holmes, 2014). Increased geographic distances may decrease connection to peers and may contribute to relaxed confidentiality practices among members.

Keeping counseling groups closed whenever possible, requiring sign-in procedures, prescreening group members, creating group rules, and reiterating those group rules can help minimize confidentiality risks and increase member comfort. Even with these precautions, DC/TMH groups are most productive when led by skilled group facilitators that can successfully navigate group process in the selected DC/TMH format.

ONLINE GROUP FACILITATION SKILLS

Facilitating DC/TMH groups requires preparation on the part of the facilitator. As discussed, practices such as reviewing informed consent, screening members, and using secure software systems with password or entry codes, lay the foundation for a successful online group. As with all DC, a detailed safety plan including emergency contacts must be on file for all clients prior to the group's commencement. Once the group is underway, there are additional strategies that the facilitator can utilize to optimize successful progress. It should be noted that best practices suggest online groups be limited to no more than six participants in order to allow for appropriate group facilitation (Kozlowski & Holmes, 2017).

Setting Boundaries and Group Rules

All effective group counseling uses some level of group rules, boundaries, or guidelines (Corey et al., 2013). Common group rules in F2F groups include putting away phones, arriving on time, not having side conversations, and minimizing crosstalk. While similar rules and boundaries exist in DC/TMH groups, they can at times be harder to enforce due to the distance between facilitator and members. It is helpful for group facilitators to review group rules and boundaries during screening and at the beginning of group meetings. For synchronous meetings, some facilitators elect to review group rules before every meeting, which can be particularly effective for telephone meetings. Others elect to post group rules in the discussion board or chat feature, either at the beginning of the session for synchronous meetings, or as a standing post for asynchronous meetings. Whichever way the counselor elects to post or share rules, it is important that group rules are reviewed regularly, and referenced when addressing behavior that violates these rules.

Group rules in online groups will vary based on the group format. For video and telephone groups, group rules may include meeting in a quiet and confidential location, turning off voice-activated recording features, minimizing distractions, and avoiding multitasking. Group rules may also involve language, such as avoiding name-calling, curses or insults, or speaking only from one's experience (e.g., keeping it in the "I") as opposed to generalizing one's experiences to an entire group.

The challenge of boundaries in online group counseling mirror those of in-person groups, such as the inability to ensure confidentiality, and the potential danger/impact of relationships outside of group. However, the digital nature of DC/TMH groups may unintentionally encourage boundary crossing. One example is searching for group members or group leaders on the Internet or via social media, then attempting to connect with group members/leaders outside of group. While this potential boundary crossing exists in F2F groups, the distance between members created by DC/TMH may contribute to curiosity and a desire for connection. In a F2F group, members often engage in small talk prior to or at the end of group. In F2F groups, members may elect to get a cup of coffee from the kitchen or go out to smoke a cigarette with peers before or after groups. When a shared interest or idea comes up in a F2F group, a member might say "we'll talk about that after group" in an effort to keep the focus on group content. In DC/TMH groups, that social interaction before and after group can be lost, both for clients and counselors (Sansom-Daly et al., 2015), which can contribute to people seeking connections via digital relationships outside of group time. While the facilitator cannot physically prevent these digital relationships, it's important that the facilitator discuss how they may impact the group dynamics. Group counseling allows members to share only what they want to share with the group, and maintain privacy in other areas of their lives. Searches such as those described violate that privacy and contribute to lack of trust among group members.

Engaging Group Members

Distance counseling groups have been found to be effective with several issues and populations (Morland et al., 2011; Sansom-Daly et al., 2015). Despite these positive outcomes, clients have reported that online groups feel artificial, too casual, as well as linear (Kozlowski & Holmes, 2014). Counselors facilitating online groups have reported difficulty balancing talk time of participants, using appropriate interventions, exploring at a deeper level, and dealing with silence (Kit et al., 2014). Kozlowski and Holmes (2017) offer a variety of strategies to the newly trained counselor who will be facilitating DC/TMH groups. They suggest that after reviewing informed consents, the first online group session should address the technology and how to utilize technology with the group. This ensures that all participants know how to use the technology and are able to do so. It is also suggested that introductions may take more time in online groups. The facilitator may elect to have members share artifacts (e.g., pictures, songs, images) that help members introduce themselves in a more personalized manner.

The online group facilitator has an active role in attempting to link client statements to one another. When online groups feel artificial, participants take on more of a "student role" and wait to be called on by the facilitator (Kozlowski & Holmes, 2014). This linear "turn taking" has the unwanted effect of some clients disengaging from the group until they are called upon to speak/write. In order to avoid these linear and artificial settings, online group facilitators work diligently to create linkages between clients' statements and experiences. This of course requires counselors to be astutely monitoring group content from all members, and making connections, either verbally or in writing, between these statements.

The facilitator's role encourages communication among group members, which can be challenging when trying to manage crosstalk. One way to facilitate this communication is to invite members to speak directly to one another; for example, the counselor can write/state, "Would someone like to respond to what [Client A] has shared?" Facilitators can also foster intergroup dialogue by redirecting clients when they speak/type to the facilitator about a client in the group. For example, the Client B starts to say, "I can relate to what [Client A] said, and I feel bad for them...." The counselor might politely interrupt and say, "I'm sorry to interrupt you, [Client B], but I'm going to ask you to speak directly to [Client A] and continue to share your thoughts." The facilitator might then encourage Client A to respond to Client B's statement, if they don't do so automatically.

Managing Talk Time and Silence

Online group facilitators have reported struggles in managing participant talk time, as well as experiencing silence (Kit et al., 2014). Much like in F2F groups, online group facilitators have to manage individuals who monopolize group time, as well as those who are disengaged and inactive. Some facilitators employ a time-sensitive model (e.g., specify minutes of talk time per each participant) yet these models may encourage linear communication, fail to foster intergroup dialogue, and reduce the immediacy and here-and-now effect of group counseling. Talk time should be addressed in group guidelines. Some common group guidelines might include statements such as "share talk time" or "everyone participates." These group rules can serve as reminders to people who monopolize or disengage, although clients may continue to display this behavior. As in F2F groups, there will be times where facilitators will need to confront monopolizing, silence, or other behaviors that impact the group process. This can be done by simply speaking/writing directly to the participant regarding the behavior. For example, when addressing monopolizers, the facilitator can state/write, "I'm going to interrupt you for a moment, Client A. While I appreciate your sharing, I'd like to hear someone else's perspective on what we are discussing." When addressing those who are disengaged, the facilitator can state/write, "We have not yet heard from you today, Client A, and I'd appreciate you sharing your thoughts on what we've discussed."

Silence during online groups can occur in any group modality, including telephone, video, or discussion boards. In DC/TMH groups, silence can be confused for dropped calls or software problems. As part of a thorough DC/TMH informed consent, protocols should be outlined for dropped or disconnected sessions. Because of these delays, it is important to instruct members that there may be a few seconds of silence after each member speaks to allow for delayed communication or processing. Group facilitators can encourage silence by inviting members to take a few moments to reflect and process what was said (Kozlowski & Holmes, 2017), and then open the floor up to member comments. In synchronous settings, such as telephone, video, and discussion boards, one member may intentionally start speaking or typing before another member finishes. It helps for the facilitator and group to agree on a signal to verify that they are done speaking. For example, in some online discussion board groups, members type the word "done" when finished. Similar systems may be devised when a person wants to speak such as a "raise hand" feature on a videoconference, or a symbol, such as an asterisk (*), to raise one's hand on a discussion board.

Ethical Guidelines

DC/TMH group facilitators must practice ethically. The Association for Specialists in Group Work (ASGW) outlines the ethical expectations for those focusing on group counseling. Specifically, ASGW publishes the *Best Practice Guidelines* (Thomas & Pender, 2008), which serves as an adjunct to the ACA's Code of Ethics. These guidelines provide direction to individuals practicing distance group counseling. Some elements of the guidelines are fundamental, such as having a primary responsibility to the group, having training to address the group need, and only practicing within their professional competence. These guidelines reiterate the counselor's need to be responsive to all clients in DC/TMH groups, as well as their responsibility to be properly trained in distance group counseling. These guidelines require facilitators to screen group members, outline participation requirements, and discuss the confidentiality limits of groups with all group members.

The ASGW Best Practices address technology by requiring that practitioners follow professional guidelines when using technology in their practice. These practices are more thoroughly outlined in the ASGW A.9: Trends and Technological Changes, which clarify how practitioners remain abreast of technological changes in areas such as practice, financial, legal, and ethical guidelines. The standards also require group practitioners to assess their population's demographic and clinical need, in determining the appropriateness of technological service delivery.

These directives recognize the role that technology plays in the provision of group counseling. More importantly the guidelines emphasize counselor's awareness of technology and remaining current on communication devices and delivery systems, such as DC/TMH group delivery. This includes an awareness of demographic and client needs, indicating that counselors should be aware of how technology may or may not be appropriate for the clients they serve.

Recognizing client needs and being responsive to those needs is central to the *ASGW Multicultural and Social Justice Competency Principles for Group Workers* (Singh et al., 2012). While technology has the ability to bring people together, socioeconomic, geographic, and disability barriers prevent certain groups from accessing that technology. Counselors delivering DC/TMH groups must consider accessibility issues when designing or delivering groups to specific populations. These principles require group facilitators to "recognize obstacles that group members encounter based on lack of opportunities and systems of oppression (e.g., sexism, classism, heterosexism) and gain awareness of how to integrate an advocacy focus into group learning to address these barriers" (Singh et al., 2012, p. 4). Additionally, these principles call on group facilitators to recognize cultural differences in communication, language, confrontation, confidentiality, and other areas, as well as to seek opportunities to incorporate mutual respect of these differences within the group. The principles instruct group facilitators to "use technology for activism and community-organizing related to group work and increasing equity through resources and access to group work" (p. 7), to emphasize their responsibility to foster social justice among the clients they serve.

CHALLENGES AND OPPORTUNITIES

The benefits of online counseling include concepts such as convenience and low cost, and the ability to access populations that normally are unable to access treatment. The benefits of group counseling include Yalom's therapeutic factors, such as universality, altruism, and catharsis (1995), among others. Yet, novice group facilitators identified the following challenges when beginning to facilitate online groups: managing resistance, managing talk time, using interventions, modeling mutual respect, achieving group goals, setting group tone, dealing with silence, confrontation, boundaries, anxiety and lack of confidence, processing in the here-and-now, and exploring issues at a deeper level (Kit et al., 2014, p. 326). Some of these challenges have been addressed already, such as managing monopolizers and unengaged individuals. Other challenges, as well as opportunities are discussed in the following.

Identity, Privacy, and Security

Using DC/TMH always requires attention to privacy and security. Concepts such as encrypted technologies, passwords, and code words are regularly utilized in DC/TMH practice. In individual DC/TMH sessions, ethics require counselors to verify client identity and confirm privacy. Recommendations for verifying identity involve showing photo ID or using code words at the beginning of session. Confirming privacy is conducted by asking the client if they are in a private location, or scanning a video device around the room if using video technology. In a group counseling setting, these practices pose some risks. Individuals may not want to expose strangers to a video scan of their home. Clients may be uncomfortable or unwilling to display a government ID on a screen with unknown peers. The use of code words in a group exposes other group members to the code word, minimizing its impact as a security/screening measure. Strategies to avoid these risks include only verifying identity during the prescreening phase of group, or having group members change code words regularly and communicate those changes to the facilitator. While these strategies may be effective for phone or video sessions, other strategies may be necessary for discussion boards.

Open groups versus closed groups pose different identity verification challenges. For online open groups, including discussion boards, conference calls, and videoconferencing, verifying identity is challenging, if not impossible based on the nature of members entering the group at any time without prescreening. On the negative side, there have been multiple reports of unknown individuals entering both video and discussion board meetings to create disruptions, such as making racist, sexual, or other inappropriate comments (Singer et al., 2020). On the positive side, online discussion boards in recovery communities allow participants to use pseudonyms, which support the anonymity of these communities (General Services Office, 2018). Closed discussion boards, where individuals sign in with a personal logon and password, serve as a mechanism for verifying identity. If individuals are provided with a log on and password by a facilitator to access a discussion forum, this may serve as verification, although it is possible that another individual has accessed the group member's information. There is also evidence to support that logging on to a secure discussion forum reinforces feelings of trust and safety among group members (Haberstroh et al., 2006). The challenges with verifying identity reinforce the recommended best practice of limiting online group counseling sessions to six people (Kozlowski & Holmes, 2017).

Larger numbers of people create greater security risks. While the counselor must take abundant precautions to utilize encryption and remove voice-activated recording devices, the counselor has limited control over the client's technology other than asking them to utilize (or not utilize) certain features. When multiple clients are involved, that control is further diminished. In individual DC/TMH sessions, the client and the counselor can discuss any desire to record sessions, which would also be outlined in an informed consent document. In some settings, recordings may be allowed for counselor training and development, or client growth and reflection. These agreements have been verified via signed release forms. In group settings, it is difficult to get all parties involved to consent to recordings. Of greater concern is that one group member may record the group without others knowing. A client who records an individual session without permission risks only their own confidentiality, yet a client who records a group without permission violates the confidentiality of everyone in that group.

Current technology allows computers and devices to easily capture recordings and images with the touch of a button. While informed consents and group rules can prohibit recording and photos, there are other protective measures. For video sessions, asking clients to sit arms distance away from their device, with their hands in view of the camera, can minimize intentional or accidental screen captures. In addition, software exists that prohibits screenshots and recordings (Dinita, 2016; Perez, 2019), although the software may not be compatible with technologies utilized for online groups. For discussion boards, regular reminders that prohibit recordings or photos can be posted. Members that violate these practices likely need to be removed from the group. For these reasons, as well as others, it is important that the group facilitator has a mechanism for removing an individual who is disruptive or damaging to the group dynamic.

Cross Talk

Cross talk is often discouraged in group counseling sessions, yet in online group counseling, cross talk may create a mechanism for clients to feel connected to one another. Cross talk can be described as clients talking about an unrelated topic or engaging in conversation with one another. Some group facilitators consider cross talk to be distracting from the group topic or disrespectful to either the group leader or group members. It is clear how in an online group format, such as a telephone or video conference, multiple members communicating at the same time would create a distraction. Even on discussion boards, one member may begin to type their experience before another member has finished sharing. In some discussion boards, members type an ellipsis (. . .) to indicate that they are not yet done typing, or pausing before typing again.

Online groups run the risk of becoming linear and slipping in to "turn taking" (Kozlowski & Holmes, 2014). To avoid linearity, intergroup dialogue is encouraged and facilitated by the counselor. As stated earlier, the counselor has an active role in facilitating peer-to-peer connections in an online group. Thus, cross talk may improve group member connections when conducted in a manner that respects other members of the group and the group leader. This requires the group facilitator to manage the talk time of the group, finding the delicate balance of encouraging members to speak to one another, while also holding others accountable for speaking out of turn.

Lurkers

"Lurker" refers to individuals who mostly observe and read in online group discussion boards, but rarely participate (Boniel-Nissim, 2016). Lurkers are distinguished from active participants, also known as posters (Petrovcic & Petric, 2014). Lurkers do benefit from observing in these forums, although there is evidence to support that posters benefit more from participation in online forums. Lurkers do not necessarily pose a threat to online groups, but may impact group dynamics. Other members may question lurkers commitment to the group or be mistrustful of lurkers who do not equally share in the group process. Larger groups likely contribute to more lurkers. Some discussion boards allow the facilitator and group members to see which members are "idle," meaning not actively engaged in the session. While the concept of lurkers and posters is used in relation to online discussion boards, it can be applied to participation rates of group members in other modalities, such as video or telephone conferencing. Similar to disengaged or minimally engaged group participants, lurkers can be invited to contribute to the discussion during synchronous groups.

Credibility of Posted Items

One of the benefits of online group counseling is the opportunity to share resources. Group members and leaders can share items such as images, documents, videos, and web resources. ACA (2014) ethical codes require group facilitators to ensure the quality and validity of resources that they share with their clients. However, depending on the modality, clients may be able to share items with the group that are inaccurate, inappropriate, or clinically dangerous. Even when clients are well-intentioned in sharing resources, they are not held to the same ethical standards of validating the resources they share with group members. Counselors need detailed policies for what groups members share or post in the group (Boniel-Nissim, 2016). Counselors may elect to prescreen posted items, or reserve the right to remove posted items that pose risks to clients. If the counselor elects to remove posted items, the technology must provide them with the authorization to remove items. Some counselors may elect to post items on behalf of clients once the items have been reviewed.

Safety

Distance group counseling requires detailed safety plans for every member of the group, including emergency contacts. These plans must be in place prior to the start of groups, and new members should not be able join the group until a detailed safety plan is on file. These safety plans are used when a client indicates harm to themselves or harm to others. Client safety also includes protecting group members from inaccurate, inappropriate, or clinically dangerous material, as discussed earlier. Client safety includes protecting clients from hate speech, insults, or threats from other group members. As discussed, group rules and informed consent documents can outline policies, but counselors are the vehicles by which these rules are enforced. When damaging or dangerous speech is shared in a group setting, clients will look to the counselor to respond to those comments, and reinforce group rules. Silence or lack of response to these types of remarks on the part of the counselor impacts trust and group cohesion.

CASE STUDY: ONLINE GROUP COUNSELING

Counselor A is a mental health counselor in a university counseling center. The university has a high demand for counseling services and a large commuter population. In order to meet this demand, the university has implemented synchronous online group counseling via a secure discussion board that requires students to sign on via the university portal. Counselor A runs an 8-week closed group on managing anxiety. Counselor A conducted an intake with Client 9 to address anxiety. At the end of the intake, it was suggested that Client 9 attend weekly individual sessions on campus. Client 9 reported an inability to travel to campus for weekly sessions because Client 9 no longer has access to a vehicle. Counselor A told Client 9 about the ongoing group on managing anxiety; however, since the group started 2 weeks ago, Client 9 would need to wait 6 weeks before the next session starts. Client 9 became tearful stating that they'll never get through midterms without help. Although the counseling center does not allow students to join closed groups after they start, Counselor A felt that Client 9 needed immediate support and provided her with logon information to the weekly group, explaining that she could be an observer. Below is a transcript of Client 9's first group.

DISCUSSION	PARTICIPANTS
Counselor A: The time is 8:05 PM and we will start our group. Please remember our group rules that were emailed to you before we started our group 2 weeks ago. Our topic for tonight is Coping with Anxiety Surrounding Accomplishments. If you would like to volunteer to speak, please raise your hand with an * and you will be called on. Is there anyone who would like to begin? done	Counselor A Client 1 Client 2 Client 3 Client 6 Client 7 Client 9
Client 3: *	Idle Participants Client 4 Client 8

(continued)

DISCUSSION	PARTICIPANTS

Counselor A: Go ahead Client 3. done

Client 3: Who is Client 9 and why are they here? done

Counselor A: I apologize. Tonight we are going to have an observer in the group, Client 9. She will be observing our group from now until the end of the sessions. Did you have something you wanted to share, Client 3? Done

Client 3: Nope. Not now. DONE

Counselor A: Okay. How about someone else? Would someone else like to discuss tonight's topic and how their week has been? Done
[silence]
Counselor A: I don't see any raised hands. Please type * if you'd like to share.
[silence]
Counselor A: I'm hoping we are still connected. Maybe we can just go around the room and people can tell us how their week was. Client 1, would you be willing to start and tell us either about the topic or your week? Done

Client 1: Not really but okay. My week was pretty standard. I struggle a lot with this topic and what other people want from me. . .

Client 1: Mostly around my grades and my major since I know that my paren—

Client 9: Can I say something?

Counselor A: Client 9, we don't talk out of turn in the group, but you can raise your hand and I will call on you in order. Go ahead, Client 1. Done

Client 1: It's really just my parents and their expectations. No one else really except ma

Client 9: *

Client 9: *

Client 9: *

Client 9: I'm raising my hand. Can I talk now? I want to say something about the topic.

Counselor A: Client 9, you need to wait until the person is done sharing. You will know that they are done when they type "done." I'm sorry Client 1, continue. [silence] Done. Sorry.

(continued)

DISCUSSION	PARTICIPANTS

Client 1: I was saying maybe also my siblings because they are really successful

. . .

Client 9: **************

Counselor A: Client 9, please wait until Client 1 is done

Client 9: But she stopped typing!!!! Finally ☺ ☺

Counselor A: she indicated that she was going to continue (. . .) and she had not typed done.

Client 9: This will take forever and if we are going in order then I will go LAST!!! Maybe you won't even have TIME to get to me.

Counselor A: You need to follow the group rules, Client 9, in order to be a part of the group. Client 1 please continue. done.

Client 1: NVM. done.

DISCUSSION QUESTIONS

1. Discuss the university's decision to use the discussion board format for groups. What are the pros and cons of this format? What ethical concerns do you have, if any?

2. How do you feel about Counselor A's decision to let Client 9 join the group? How might Counselor A have done things differently to improve the outcome?

3. Consider the other members of the group. How was their engagement in the group? What hindered their engagement? What could have helped?

4. Discuss how Client 9's behavior impacted other members of the group. How did Counselor A manage the disruptions? What could they have done differently?

5. Assuming good intent, what did Counselor A do well?

CRITICAL QUESTIONS IN DECIDING TO PRACTICE

Facilitating DC/TMH groups requires skill and attention, as well as a commitment to the group process and growth. While facilitating any counseling group requires skill, consider the following elements in deciding how you would facilitate a DC/TMH group.

1. How are your group facilitation skills for in-person groups? What type of group facilitator do you think you are?

2. What type of group are you planning to run? Psychoeducation, psychotherapy, other? Open or closed? What modality (telephone, video, etc.) will you use?

3. How will you prescreen your group members? How can you use that prescreening to verify identity? Do you have a DC/TMH informed consent document that includes a safety plan?

4. What type of group rules would you establish, and when would you share them with group members? Would group members have any input on the group rules?

5. How would you facilitate intergroup dialogue among group members? What strategies would you use to help members connect with other members, while minimizing distractions?

6. How is your attention to detail, memory, and listening skills? Can you pick up on small details or nuances that connect clients to one another—and articulate those connections to clients in your group?

7. How are your confrontation skills? How do you feel about having to manage talk time, or confront clients for inappropriate behavior?

8. What mechanism would you use to remove disruptive members?

9. How might you attempt to involve lurkers or unengaged members?

10. What policies would you create for members posting information or sharing resources with the group?

VOICES FROM THE FIELD

Transitioning to Telemental Health Groups

Ryan Poole, Second Year Graduate Student, Clinical Mental Health Counseling

I was enrolled in an internship at a local substance abuse facility where I regularly participated in group sessions. As a result of the COVID-19 closure, after receiving telemental health training, I transitioned to providing videoconferencing psychoeducational groups on stress management for other graduate students at my institution. From my perspective, the main change in the transition would be that I was not able to do small things to encourage participation during the online group. In an in-person group, I could make eye contact with the entire group; or if someone hasn't spoken yet in a group, I would use nonverbals and reassurances toward them. This was my way of encouraging them to speak, and subtly telling them that I know they haven't contributed, without saying a word. If that failed, I would just outright ask them for their perspective. However, I feel I have to utilize "callouts" more often in the online group. Furthermore, I would say group participation is lower in the online group. Seeing people in person during group is much different than on camera. I believe it is easy for people to feel lost in the shuffle and that makes them not want to participate.

Another difference I became aware of was the attitudes and behaviors of group members. In a group setting at a treatment facility, most people have had to shower, groom, and eaten something before attending a group. Furthermore, if they showed up to group at a treatment facility in pajamas or looking like a mess you would naturally confront them about it. In the telemental health environment, people can realistically wake up just in time for the group session (and sometimes it shows). The main difference here is attitude. A person who went through their entire routine and braved the world before going to treatment is going to be ready to start exploring themselves in group versus someone who has been home. For those that have been home, it is usually a bit slow to get them to come along and be active participants.

Finally, at the treatment facility, the group was about maintaining sobriety. This is an essential tool for the functioning of the group members. Due to emphasis on functioning, most clients come in ready to discuss aspects of their life, small to large. In the telemental health group, the focus was nonessential. Our group was optional for graduate students. Since people come in with the attitude that the group was optional, I shouldn't be shocked that getting more participation from them was difficult. I am sad that my internship site does not have the infrastructure for telemental health groups because I'm sure I would be able to notice more nuances and subtler things. Because this was such a huge change, I wonder how much my observations are based solely on subject matter or the change of group members.

CONCLUSION

Group counseling encompasses many types of groups including task/working groups, psychoeducation groups, counseling groups, psychotherapy groups, or mixed groups. Counseling groups are composed of group dynamic which include both the group content and the group process. All types of groups may utilize DC or TMH via multiple modalities including videoconferencing, telephone, chatrooms, and synchronous or asynchronous discussion boards. Like F2F groups, DC/TMH groups may be open or closed, and rely on trust among group members and the group facilitator. Managing group dynamics in a DC/TMH group can be challenging and the counselor must be prepared to set boundaries and enforce group rules. Counselors must try to engage group members, manage talk time among members, and navigate silence, which can be challenging in spoken or typed settings. Group distance counselors follow ethical guidelines, such as those established by the ASGW. Like F2F groups, counselors must explain issues of confidentiality and privacy, while also addressing issues such as technological security and verifying identity. Distance group counselors need to manage crosstalk, ensure that items shared are credible, and manage client safety via detailed procedures and planning.

REFERENCES

Alcoholics Anonymous. (2020). *Over 80 years of growth*. Timeline view. https://www.aa.org/pages/en_US/aa-timeline/to/1

American Counseling Association. (2014). *2014 code of ethics*. https://www.counseling.org/resources/aca-code-of-ethics.pdf

Boniel-Nissim, M. (2016). Using forums to enhance client peer support. In S. Goss, K. Anthony, L. Sykes Stretch, & D. Merz Nagel (Eds.), *Technology in mental health: Applications in practice, supervision, and training*. Charles C. Thomas Publishers.

Corey, M. S., Corey, G., & Corey, C. (2013). *Groups: Process and practice* (9th ed.). Brooks/Cole.

Dinita, M. (2016, November 16). *3 best anti-screenshot software for Windows 10*. Windows Report. https://windowsreport.com/anti-screen-capture-software

General Services Office. (2018). *A.A. guidelines: Internet*. https://www.aa.org/assets/en_US/mg-18_internet.pdf

Gladding, S. T. (2012). *Groups: A counseling specialty* (6th ed.). Pearson.

Haberstroh, S., Parr, G., Gee, R., & Trepal, H. (2006). Interactive e-journaling in group work: Perspectives from counselor trainees. *The Journal for Specialists in Group Work, 31*, 327–337. https://doi.org/10.1080/01933920600918840

In the Rooms. (2020). *About us*. https://www.intherooms.com/home/about-in-the-rooms

Kit, P. L., Wong, S. S., D-Rozario, V., & Teo, C. T. (2014). Exploratory findings on novice group counselors' initial co-facilitating experiences in in-class support groups with adjunct online support groups. *The Journal for Specialists in Group Work, 39*, 316–344. https://doi.org/10.1080/01933922.2014.954737

Kozlowski, K. A., & Holmes, C. M. (2014). Experiences in online process groups: A qualitative study. *Journal for Specialists in Group Work, 39*, 276–300. https://doi.org/10.1080/01933922.2014.948235

Kozlowski, K. A., & Holmes, C. M. (2017). Teaching online group counseling skills in an on campus group counseling course. *The Journal of Counselor Preparation and Supervision, 9*(1). https://doi.org/10.7729/91.1157

Morland, L. A., Hynes, A. K., Mackintosh, M-A., Resick, P. A., & Chard, K. M. (2011). Group cognitive processing therapy delivered to veterans via telehealth: A pilot cohort. *Journal of Traumatic Stress, 24,* 465–469.

Perez, S. (2019, May 16). Ticketmaster puts an end to screenshots with new digital ticket technology. *Tech Crunch.* https://techcrunch.com/2019/05/16/ticketmaster-put-an-end-to-screenshots-with-new-digital-ticket-technology

Petrovcic, A., & Petric, G. (2014). Differences in intrapersonal and interactional empowerment between lurkers and posters in health-related online support communities. *Computers in Human Behavior, 34,* 39–28. https://dx.doi.org/10.1016/j.chb.2014.01.008

Sansom-Daly, U. M., Wakefield, C. E., McGill, B. C., & Patterson, P. (2015). Ethical and clinical challenges delivering group-based cognitive-behavioural therapy to adolescents and young adults with cancer using videoconferencing technology. *Australian Psychologist, 50,* 271–278.

Singer, N., Perlroth, N., & Krolik, A. (2020, April 8). Zoom rushes to improve privacy for consumers flooding its service. *New York Times.* https://www.nytimes.com/2020/04/08/business/zoom-video-privacy-security-coronavirus.html

Singh, A. A., Merchant, N., Skudrzyk, B., & Ingene, D. (2012). *Association for Specialists in Group Work: Multicultural and Social Justice Competence Principles for Group Workers.* https://www.asgw.org/resources-1

Thomas, R. V., & Pender, D. A. (2008). Association for specialists in group work: Best practice guidelines 2007 revisions. *The Journal for Specialists in Group Work, 33,* 111–117. https://doi.org/10.1080/01933920801971184

Yalom, I. D. (1995). *Theory and practice of group psychotherapy* (4th ed.). Basic Books Inc.

7

Career Development and Telemental Health

INTRODUCTION

Technology has become a critical component of distance career service delivery. These distance modalities include, but are not limited to, telephone, videoconferencing, text, email, chatrooms, and self-contained platforms incorporating multiple modalities. Within the mental health realm, these services are referred to as telemental health (TMH). However, distance services are not confined to those providing mental health counseling. A wide variety of career practitioners utilize distance counseling. The most recent Code of Ethics of the National Career Development Association (NCDA) and the National Employment Counseling Association's (NECA) Employment Counseling Competencies (2001) include both technology and computer use with clients. These ethical changes demonstrate the growing use of technology in career services. Career development encompasses a variety of services including career information, career guidance, career assessment, and career counseling. These distinctions help classify the type of services that are provided via distance counseling (DC). In addition, these services can be provided in either self-help or counselor-supported formats. While there are a variety of benefits to online career services, there are equal concerns about the quality and validity of these services (Sampson & Makela, 2014).

Delivering career services via the Internet is not a new phenomenon. Published guides on delivering career services via the Internet have been available for over a decade (Mulcahy Boer, 2009). Despite the longevity of distance career services, practitioners hesitate to engage in this practice or seek additional information before doing so. This hesitancy may be based on practitioners' views of online services as a replacement, alternative, or substitute for counselor-led services (Bright, 2015). Additionally, individuals or organizations may be unready or unwilling to engage in distance practices (Harris-Bowlsbey & Sampson, 2005). A final concern may be a need for training in distance career services (Harris-Bowlsbey & Sampson, 2005; Venable, 2010). This chapter outlines the benefits and cautions of distance career service delivery in order to aid the practitioner in the decision to adapt their career practice to distance modalities.

GROWTH OF CAREER SERVICES ONLINE

One of the earliest organized counseling services in the United States is known to be Frank Parsons's Breadwinner's Institute, developed in 1905, to assist young men with their job and career options. Parsons went on to publish *Choosing a Vocation* in 1909, becoming known as the Father of Vocational Guidance (Brown, 2016). Career counseling is recognized as one of the first counseling specializations and has a long history in the United States. Beginning in the 1960s, career counseling was also one of the first specializations to utilize computer-automated guidance systems (CAGS) and computer information guidance systems (CIGS) to provide services to clients (Brown, 2016). Career services' early adoption of technology was driven largely by the growing and changing nature of the workforce, as well as the availability of career information (Harris-Bowlsbey & Sampson, 2005).

The United States Bureau of Labor Statistics (BLS) began collecting employment and industry data in the 1910s and published the first Occupational Outlook Handbook (OOH) in 1949 (BLS, 2019). The Dictionary of Occupational Titles (DOT) was published in 1939 (Brown, 2016). Information gathered by the BLS and published in the DOT and OOH is known as labor market information (LMI). As the workforce continued to evolve, computer software systems provided a mechanism for counselors and clients to store and retrieve vast amounts of LMI on a multitude of careers. In the 1970s the Department of Labor provided funding to 23 states to create career information systems for students and young adults. These projects corresponded with several legislative measures in the 1970s to increase education and employment options (Jacobson & Grabowski, 1981). In 1994, the DOT began transitioning to the O*Net online, and the transition was completed in 2001. The OOH began transitioning online in 1996 and was an online only publication by 2011 (BLS, 2019). Around this same time period, paper and pencil career assessments were moved to computer scoring and online administration (Osborn et al., 2019). As more career information moved to online spaces, more career practitioners began using online tools with their students and clients.

DEFINING DISTANCE CAREER SERVICES

Consider the myriad of services that career professionals provide, including counseling, coaching, intake, assessment, career information delivery, education, skill development, and others. It is necessary to define distance career services, such that our clients are able to identify quality services and counselors are able to practice ethically. The NCDA serves practitioners and educators who assist individuals to achieve satisfying career and life outcomes. The NCDA defines the roles of career planning and career counseling in their Code of Ethics. Career planning services provide information to assist with a specific client outcome, which may include needs related to their job search or career decision-making process (NCDA, 2015a). Career counseling is a counseling relationship in which the client and counselor establish a professional rapport and explore more significant issues related to career and personal goals (NCDA, 2015a). The NCDA specifies that all career practitioners work only in areas that are suited for their professional training and expertise. This NCDA distinction between career planning and career counseling begins to address one of the challenges of providing career services online; specifically, what are the credentials of the provider and what are they qualified to provide? This concern will be addressed later in this chapter under "Challenges and Opportunities."

Providing career information is another function of a career practitioner (Kettunen et al., 2015). The NCDA defines career information as "either given or received. Information may be fact or opinion, valid or invalid, simple or complex, current or outdated, presented in or out of context, useful or not useful. The information itself is a tool" (NCDA, 2015b, p. 4). This NCDA definition of career information highlights an additional challenge of distance career services. Career practitioners regularly provide career information online, both to the clients they serve and to the public. New technologies allow individuals to put out information on career development, or any other topic, with relative ease. Some examples include buying a domain name and creating a website, publishing a blog, video, or podcast, sending information via a listserv, or posting information on social media sites, such as Twitter, LinkedIn, and Facebook. Individuals can post whatever they like without much oversight or verification. How does the public know what is trustworthy career information? How can counselors be sure that the career information they provide to clients is ethical, reliable, valid, and accurate?

PROVIDING DISTANCE CAREER DEVELOPMENT

The NCDA Code of Ethics (2015a) provides guidance to the distance career counselor. In this chapter, specific sections of the NCDA code are indicated in parentheses. First, counselors must have expertise in providing distance services (F1a). They must be aware of state laws and statutes pertaining to distance services (F1b). While laws and statutes will vary from state to state, it is the counselor's responsibility to be knowledgeable of these laws/statutes. Second, counselors must create detailed informed consent and disclosure policies (F2a). These statements and policies must address confidentiality and its limits (F2b). Counselors must also ensure that their online practice utilizes privacy protections and encryptions (F2c).

Counselors engaging in distance career services must verify client identity throughout the counseling relationship (F3). Because of the nature of distance services and the absence of face-to-face (F2F) contact, the counselor must verify that the person being communicated with via phone, text, or email, is truly the intended client. Client verification is completed initially by requesting government issued photo ID, and then conducting an in-person or video session to verify that identity. For text, email, or phone sessions, client identity is verified by using code words or a communication pattern which is only known to the client and counselor (NCDA, 2015a). Finally, a comprehensive intake should be conducted to include emergency contacts and an emergency plan. This includes a plan for verifying the client's physical location at the beginning of each session. Should emergency personnel need to be contacted, the counselor must be able to accurately report on the client's location. Most importantly, determining if the client is the right fit for distance counseling is critical. The client must have the cognitive, emotional, and technical ability to navigate distance communication and handle any potential challenges that may arise when using technology for career services.

Career Counseling

An important step for any career professional is to carefully consider what services they will provide and ensure that they are qualified to provide those services. As the NCDA definition specifies, there is a clear distinction between career planning and career counseling. Individuals who provide online career services must accurately advertise the services they will provide, and ensure that they have expertise in career development *and* distance delivery. While there is currently no state license for a career counselor, there are national credentials such as the Global Career Development Facilitator (GCDF) or the NCDA credentials, such as the Master Career Services Professional (MCSP), that signify expertise in career development. Certificates are also available in distance counseling practice, known as telemental health (TMH) or telehealth. Best practices suggest that those who provide online career services accurately post their credentials and their expertise in career development and distance delivery. The NCDA codes specify that counselors seek expertise and assistance on technical issues, particularly those that cross state lines or international boundaries (F1c).

Career counseling requires a professional relationship, trust, and rapport with the client. When services are delivered in a distance format, counselors are responsible for educating clients on the differences in electronic communication (F4e). Clients or counselors may misinterpret verbal or nonverbal communication. Lack of body language and facial expressions impacts how clients interpret information. In a F2F session, nonverbal communication would signal if the client was overwhelmed or confused. In distance sessions, counselors need to check in with clients regularly regarding their thoughts or feelings. Silence or delays in response time may be due to technology, or may be used intentionally by client or counselor. For video sessions, slow bandwidth may cause sessions to lag. It may be difficult to tell when a client has stopped speaking or typing, and practitioners may unintentionally interrupt clients. Video images may freeze while audio communication continues. Eye contact may appear diverted as counselors usually look at the client on screen during sessions as opposed to looking at the camera. As a result, counselors appear to be looking down, instead of at the client. This can be addressed by relocating the client image to appear directly below the camera and moving the practitioner's gaze closer to the top of the screen. Portraying and interpreting emotion can be challenging. Videoconferencing and telephone conferencing allow the counselor to hear or see some emotional response. Yet services such as text, chat, and email present obstacles in recognizing emotion. Elements of the typed word, such as responding in all capital letters, excessive or limited use of punctuation, use of text grammar, and emoticons may complicate communication. It is recommended that counselors develop their own guidelines and protocols, or develop these protocols with clients, in order to avoid misinterpretation of emotion or intent. Counselors must communicate these potential problems (F4e), ask clients their preference, and adapt their style to suit the client's comfort level.

Career Assessment

Career assessments delivered in a computer-based or online format are referred to as computer-assisted career assessments (CACA; Osborn et al., 2019). There is debate as to what constitutes a CACA. While people traditionally consider career assessments to measure traits such as abilities, interests, or values (NCDA, 2015a), a CACA may include a digital slideshow reflecting a student's career interests or a video portfolio of one's career skills (Osborn et al., 2019). Career assessments have the ability to be completed independently or with the support of a counselor. Self-help assessments are available to the public online, or may be facilitated by a counselor providing access to an instrument.

The benefits of CACAs include ease of client access, simplified storing of results, simplified scoring, as well as personalized reports. Scoring and interpretation is fast, and results are easily shared with the client. Assessment results can be linked to a vast amount of career information available online (Osborn et al., 2019). The limitations of CACAs include the cost of administering tools, as well as issues of access. Administration and scoring fees may place CACAs out of reach for some members of the public. In addition, access to computer systems, software, and the Internet is also required. There are also concerns about the quality and variety of career assessments available online. It is impossible to assess the psychometric properties of online instruments if psychometric properties are not published. Other risks include not being able to explain/support the client during administration, as well as difficulty storing and maintaining confidential information. With online, self-directed assessments, there may be advertisements or product promotion connected to assessment results (Osborn et al., 2019).

Ethical standards pertaining to in-person career assessments also apply to online career assessments. For example, counselor competence, appropriate use, informed consent, awareness of cultural sensitivity and historical prejudice, and issues with diagnoses all must be considered when administering assessments in-person or online. Regardless of in-person or online administration, counselors are responsible for being trained to both administer and interpret results, maintain security of results, refrain from using outdated instruments, and obtain client consent for assessment (NCDA, Section E, 2015a). There are specific guidelines for counselors administering CACAs. First and foremost, section F4f specifies that practitioners must determine if the psychometric properties of an assessment were evaluated for online administration. This means that the reliability and validity findings from print career assessments cannot simply be transferred to online administration. Career instruments must have been tested for reliability and validity in electronic format in order for the electronic version to be reliable and valid. Counselors are required to determine if the assessment is designed for self-help or for counselor-facilitated interpretation. Counselors must maintain confidentiality of assessment results. Finally, counselors are required to refer a client to a qualified career practitioner in the client's area if it is apparent that the client is not comprehending the career assessment results delivered via distance format (NCDA, 2015a).

Career Information

The O*Net Online and the OOH are two of the most utilized, valid, and reputable resources for online career information in the United States. Published by the U.S. Department of Labor, the O*Net and OOH contain reliable information for counselors and consumers on careers, LMI, and employment trends. Additionally, features on O*Net such as My Next Move and the O*Net Interest Profiler, provide valid interest inventories based on John Holland's Theory of Vocational Guidance. Other trustworthy online career information sites include state career websites. Some examples include Career Zone, used by states such as New York, Pennsylvania, and California. While the OOH, O*Net, and state websites provide reliable information, there is doubt that these government websites will be able to produce career information systems at the same rate as the private sector, and with the level of individualism and flexibility that private sector sites provide (Bright, 2015). However, counselors need to use caution in recommending, referring, or utilizing web sources to ensure that these sites are valid and reliable. Similar to unauthorized assessments, career information websites from less reliable sources may be linked to advertisements or market research.

The NCDA Ethical Codes provide useful guidelines regarding career information. Career counselors can begin by posting accurate information about themselves and their credentials. The NCDA (F.6.c and F.7.c) requires that counselors disclose not only their own qualifications, but the qualifications of the individual providing the career information content. This means that when counselors elect to post or share information with their clients or the public, they ensure that the author of those materials is qualified to provide career information. In addition, accurate sources and citations must be provided for information that is posted or shared. When the credentials and/or sources of career information are not valid, counselors refrain from sharing information with their clients or the public that may be inaccurate or incomplete. Counselors select reputable and reliable sources of information, such as government websites and peer-reviewed journal articles.

Counselors avoid recommending sites or resources that present a conflict of interest; for example, when a career counselor co-created a career assessment and receives a payment every time a client takes this assessment. When working with clients, the counselor would want to expose clients to a wide variety of career assessments available, including those that are free. If a counselor were to instruct clients to exclusively complete their assessment (unless included in your original fees/agreement), this would create a conflict of interest. Similarly, imagine a career practitioner's partner worked on commission at a business attire retail store. If that practitioner were to send all of their clients to that store to buy interview attire and instruct them to ask for their partner, this would create a conflict of interest.

Career counselors are responsible for knowing what career information is online and how it may help the clients they serve. They ensure that the career information they refer clients to is "current, valid, and free from bias" (NCDA, 2015b, p. 6). They present information to clients in a way that is easy to understand. For example, the O*Net has a wealth of information, yet can be overwhelming to visitors not familiar with the site. We often sit down with clients to explain these systems in F2F sessions. In distance sessions, counselors should employ strategies to assist the client in processing career information. Examples include using the "share screen" features of video conferencing software, video tutorials, or conducting a telephone "walk through" with the client while simultaneously reviewing career information. In these settings, clients can ask questions, receive guidance, and thoroughly understand the career information provided.

Social Media

Career counselors are required to provide career information to clients about social media and its potential impact on one's career. The NCDA (F.7.j., Educating Clients About the Role of Social Media in the Career Development Process) states that counselors will explain the role of social media in career development, including the pros and cons of using social media in the job search process (2015a). In their personal lives, and even professional roles, career counselors may elect to avoid social media, not use social media, or not discuss social media with clients. Yet because of both the risks and benefits of social media on the career search, career counselors are required to have competent understanding of social media in relation to career development.

The benefits of social media include a vast expanse of networking connections. The social media site, LinkedIn, for example, is specifically aimed at professional and career development networking. Benefits include connecting with "interest" groups, reviewing job postings available through social media platforms, or finding connections with desired employers. Others include being able to post a resume or a skill set online, which attracts recruiters, potential job prospects, or simply professional development connections. Clients may elect to put their LinkedIn profile directly on their resume, in order to demonstrate a wider variety of skills to prospective employers.

The primary risk of social media in relation to career development is the public nature of information posted. Individuals may have posted statements, pictures, or other items on social media sites that are able to be viewed by an employer based on the public nature of these sites. These posts provide an opportunity for employer judgment or discrimination, regardless of job qualifications or candidacy. Employers screen out candidates based on judgments made on the candidate's social media posts prior to making a job offer. Employers may elect to not interview a candidate based on information they review on social media. Employers may judge the activities that a client engages in, photos that they post, groups that they are affiliated with, or simply how they look and portray themselves online. This type of discrimination is difficult to detect based on the public nature of social media.

CHALLENGES AND OPPORTUNITIES

The wealth of career information and resources available online appear to support the counselor engaging in distance career counseling. Nevertheless, there are multiple challenges and cautions for both the counselor and the public to consider.

Credentialing

Earlier in this chapter you read how the NCDA created distinct definitions for career planning and career counseling. If you have read the NCDA Code of Ethics, you may have noted that the code uses the term "career professionals," as opposed to "career counselors." This is because a degree in counseling is not required to conduct career development services. In fact, many individuals with advanced degrees in Education, Human Resources, Business, and other specialties provide career services to students and adults alike. On one hand, this creates a benefit to both the consumer and the provider; more degree options allow more professionals to enter the field and provide a wider range of career services to serve the public. On the other hand, there is not necessarily a standardized education or training program for professionals in the field. While there are well-regarded certificate programs, such as the Global Career Development Facilitator (GCDF) and the NCDA career credentials, they are optional. Providers are not required to earn these credentials in order to practice. Similarly, because career concerns cannot specifically be billed to insurance, individuals seeking private career counseling often pay out of pocket. There is a risk that unqualified individuals may be providing career services, or charging inappropriate fees, due to the lack of oversight.

This lack of oversight is a problem both for in-person and distance career services, but it has unique significance for distance services. In other counseling specialties, such as mental health counseling, state licensing laws limit who can practice across state lines. For example, a counselor who is licensed in New York is not able to see clients in California, even via distance counseling, unless they obtain a license from California, and even then, may require additional protocols. California has regulations for mental health counselors that are not required in New York, such as courses on crisis counseling and marriage and family therapy. State licensing boards also provide oversight on the counselor's education, credentials, and continuing education, and receive ethics complaints on licensed providers. Due to the variable and optional credentialing standards, career practitioners with different levels of credentials are free to practice across state lines with little oversight regarding education, experiences, and complaint procedures.

Counselors wishing to practice distance career counseling can mitigate these public risks by posting their credentials and experience in career counseling, providing a grievance/complaint procedure, and seeking voluntary certifications that demonstrate career competence. Earning a professional credential such as the GCDF or NCDA's Certified Career Counselor (CCC) or Certified Master Career Specialist (CMCS), signals to the public that the provider abides by ethical codes and guidelines. The career practitioner can publish these guidelines for clients, along with links to ethics boards and complaint procedures. Joining professional organizations such as the NCDA or NECA will also provide the practitioner with up to date resources on career development practices, and reinforce their commitment to ethical practice.

Ethical Codes and Social Media

Social media has received a great deal of attention, both for its ability to connect people, but also as a forum for open-access communication. People often have multiple social media platforms that they check or post to multiple times per day. Some social media sites, such as LinkedIn, serve as a networking site and have a reputation for assisting individuals with their professional goals and career aspirations. Social media sites may be monitored by prospective or current employers. Clients have the flexibility to use these social medial sites as they wish,; for the career counselor providing distance services, however, there are cautions for its use. Interestingly, the American Counseling Association (ACA) and the NCDA vary in their ethical codes regarding social media. While the majority of the codes mirror each other, social media is one area in which the codes differ. This is significant because NECA's (2001) competencies for career professionals require adherence to the ACA code, while the NCDA publishes their own codes.

Career professionals will have to engage in personal decision-making after carefully considering the codes of both the ACA and the NCDA. For example, the ACA code of ethics (A.5.e) states that counselors may not engage in any personal relationships, including virtual relationships, with any person that they are currently counseling (ACA, 2014). This standard is not present in the NCDA code. Instead NCDA Section F.7.g, Social Media Policies and Fair and Equitable Treatment, emphasizes that career professionals create social media policies that benefit each client equally and fairly, and that these policies are equitably applied to all clients (NCDA, 2015a). The definition is expanded to provide examples of types of policies that may be created, such as no social networking connections with any clients permitted versus social network connections allowed on one specific platform. Thus, while the ACA prohibits connecting with clients via social media, the NCDA leaves it up to the organization to determine equitable policies. Neither organization advocates for career services to be offered via social media platforms, as these platforms rarely offer the security and encryption required to deliver distance services.

The NCDA provides additional guidelines not specifically outlined in the ACA code. The NCDA specifically cites the Health Insurance Portability and Accountability Act (HIPAA) and Federal Education Rights and Privacy Act (FERPA) as federal privacy guidelines (F.7.d.). The NCDA also includes provisions for respecting copyrights and original sources (F.7.i), noting the permanence and accuracy of information posted via social media (F.7.h), and educating clients about the potential impact of social media on career development (F.7.j). Both the ACA (H.6.a.) and the NCDA (F.7.b) require that practitioners keep separate personal and professional social media pages if they are using social media for professional purposes. Both the NCDA (F.7.f) and the ACA (H.6.b) require social media policies to be outlined in an informed consent document, while also requiring the practitioner to keep client information private and avoid disclosing confidential information via social media.

Access Issues

Technology is common in our society. Americans are regularly asking for the WiFi password in public places, looking for places to plug in, asking to process and pay for transactions online, and generally assuming that everyone has access to the Internet. But do they? According to a United Nations (2018) report, a little more than half of the global citizenship was using the Internet at the end of 2018. The percentage of people accessing the Internet is greater in more developed nations, such as Europe (approximately 80%) and the Americas (approximately 70%), and quickly rising in less-developed regions, such as Africa (approximately 24%). In 2019, 96% of Americans owned a cellphone. Eighty-one percent owned a smartphone, a significant increase from 35% of smartphone users in 2011 (Pew Research Group, 2019). Despite these numbers, the same U.N. report indicates that certain communities remain offline entirely. Certain demographic groups are less likely to be online, such as women and girls, the elderly, those with disabilities, indigenous populations, and those living in poverty (U.N., 2018, para. 6). Career practitioners must balance their desire to practice online with the public's access to online services. This is particularly relevant for those seeking to work with marginalized groups, including those already mentioned herein.

Counselors can begin by assessing Internet and telephone access among the populations they wish to serve. The NCDA (F.2.b) specifies the need to provide services that are accessible to persons with disabilities (PWD). The Americans with Disabilities Act website, managed by the United States Department of Justice, Civil Rights Division, publishes guidelines for websites in order to be compliant with the American with Disabilities Act (ADA, 2003). In addition, counselors should consider the multicultural and diversity needs of the community they serve (NCDA, B1a). This may be more challenging when providing online services across a vast geographic region. The NCDA and the ACA specify the need for translation services when feasible. Consider the multitude of career information online. As discussed, it is the career counselor's responsibility to ensure that career information sites used in distance practice are valid and reliable. Those sites should also be ADA compliant. For non-English speakers, that information would need to be reliably translated. Currently, the O*Net's career exploration program, My Next Move, is offered in Spanish: Mi Proximo Paso (www.miproximopaso.org). When unable to provide appropriate services, counselors provide referral assistance in locating qualified providers, which may include F2F providers. As discussed, individuals must also be appropriate for distance services, including their cognitive and developmental functioning, and ability to access the technology.

Fees

Determining fees for career development services is certainly an opportunity and a challenge. On one hand, counselors may view providing career services (either in person or online) as an opportunity to increase revenue and assist more clients, particularly with the lack of state regulations for career counseling. On the other, career counseling concerns cannot be billed to the client's insurance, unless accompanying another mental health condition such as anxiety or depression. This is because mental health counseling utilizes a medical model in which the insurance claim must be connected to a mental health diagnosis. The most common career concerns would not in and of themselves constitute a mental health diagnosis. As a result, the career practitioner is required to determine fees for their services. In most cases, the fees will be paid out of pocket, unless the client is receiving services from a local One Stop, state Vocational Rehabilitation agency, school, or college, in which case the cost of services is covered by the government, tuition, or a combination of other sources.

Determining fees can be challenging based on the type of client one is seeing, ranging from the unemployed and underemployed to the senior executive seeking a promotion or a career change. The NCDA (A9b) requires that counselors consider the financial stress of clients when setting fees. Counselors also help clients find other services at an appropriate cost if fees are not acceptable. Finding other services for clients presents an opportunity to connect clients to the vast amount of free information online, as well as their local One Stop center for F2F services. More specifically, th NCDA encourages career professionals to support their communities by providing their services pro bono or for reduced financial fees (NCDA, 2015a).

Career assessments and CACA also create challenges and opportunities regarding fees. A variety of career assessments and CAGS are available for a fee. Career practitioners who use those systems will likely need to pass those fees on to their clients and students, or require them to pay an assessment fee. Counselors need to determine if these assessments and fees are necessary. In addition, career counselors should determine if there is another, equally appropriate assessment that is offered at a reduced cost or for free, such as the O*Net's Interest Profiler or Ability Profiler.

Self-Help Versus Counselor-Facilitated

As with other areas of DC and TMH practice, there is a question as to whether online services should be self-directed or counselor facilitated. Bright (2015) argues that online career services need not engage in this either/or dichotomy, but can supplement in-person services or stand alone. Yet with the immersion of online video platforms such as YouTube, self-directed learning is on the rise. Should counselors bill for career services when so much information is available online for free? Many tasks that traditionally have been practiced or modeled with a live counselor (e.g., interviewing, resume writing, cover letter writing), are now learned via online information and videos. What is lacking with these learning systems, for the most part, is the personalized feedback. Returning to the definitions of career planning and career counseling, it is possible that while a multitude of information for career planning is available online, the feedback required for more personalized career planning requires counselor facilitation.

CASE STUDY: CAREER DEVELOPMENT

Counselor A has been providing career advising services in a college career office for the past 5 years. Counselor A has a master's degree in Education and recently completed online training to earn a Global Career Development Facilitator (GCDF) credential. Counselor A is also a member of NECA. Couselor A posted their experience, credentials, and links to GCDF and NECA complaint procedures on their website. Counselor A has decided to create an online career services business aimed specifically at new college graduates. Counselor A created a website and promoted their website through their social media contacts. Because Counselor A wanted to demonstrate their expertise in college career counseling, they used their personal Facebook and LinkedIn accounts, which document their history of working with college students. They also used an alumni email list from their employer to market their business. They use the laptop that their employer provides for all of their private online work.

Counselor A has access to a wide variety of resources through the job at the college. Specifically, Counselor A has provided private clients with career assessments that were obtained from the college office. While Counselor A has not provided their private clients with any college log-on information, they have used their college access to proprietary systems when assisting their private clients online. For example, Counselor A will utilize the "share screen" feature when conducting a videoconference session, and then use their own sign-on information to access the college systems. Through these systems, Counselor A's private clients can research employer information and see potential job opportunities that were posted for students and alumni of the college where Counselor A works. Because Counselor A knows that navigating career websites can be confusing, Counselor A allows their potential clients to record sessions such that clients can review the videos to help refresh their memory on how to navigate these websites.

Counselor A has been providing private career services online for approximately 6 months. One of the private clients they have been seeing online, Client B, was scheduled for a promising interview with a desired employer during the morning. When Counselor A had a video session with Client B that same afternoon to see how the job interview went, they were surprised by what they saw on the screen. Unlike prior sessions where Client B had been neatly dressed and seated at their desk, during today's session, Client B was lying in bed, wearing pajamas, and sobbing. They were accessing the video software from their phone as opposed to their laptop. Client B explained that they had missed their interview due to drinking the night before and slept through the interview. Client B stated that they "always do this" and that they "hate myself for screwing up again." Counselor A did not have any history on Client B's substance use history prior to this session. Counselor A notices a variety of alcohol bottles around the client and is unsure how to proceed.

DISCUSSION QUESTIONS

1. Consider the NECA code of ethics that Counselor A follows. How might their actions support or violate those codes?

2. Discuss Counselor A's use of work equipment and material to serve their personal clients. How might this violate ethical, professional, or moral codes?

3. Consider the case of Client B. What precautions should Counselor A have put in place prior to this incident?

4. Now that this incident has occurred, if you were Counselor A, how would you proceed?

5. Assuming good intentions, what did Counselor A do well, or attempt to do well?

CRITICAL QUESTIONS IN DECIDING TO PRACTICE

Are you a career counselor considering online practice? Are you an online practitioner considering branching into career development? Here are some reflection questions to consider:

1. What is your training and background in career development? If you have a master's degree in counseling, beyond the standard Career Development course you took as part of your degree, what additional training or experience do you have with career development services? Describe how career development is or has become your expertise.

2. Do you currently hold a career credential, such as the Global Career Development Facilitator (GCDF) or an NCDA career credential such as the Certified Career Counselor, or other degree? If not, are you willing to pursue/earn one?

3. What experience and training do you have providing distance services, if any? What are you willing to do to expand your DC skills, if needed?

4. What services would you offer? Career information, career guidance, career assessment, career counseling, or others? Which are you qualified to provide?

5. What professional development organizations do you belong to? Whose ethical codes do you abide by? How would you make a complaint procedure available to your clients?

6. How comfortable are you with social media? How confident would you be in advising your clients on the pros and cons of social media in the career development process? What policies would you create regarding social media?

7. Knowing that you can't bill insurance for career concerns, how would you structure your pay rates for career services? What variations would you make, say, for an executive seeking a career change versus an unemployed single parent or a new college graduate, if any? To what extent are you willing to provide pro bono or sliding scale services, if at all?

8. What online career resources would you utilize? How would you determine if they were evidence-based and reputable? How would you share the rating/reputation of these sources with your clients?

9. What type of online career assessments would you use? How would you determine if they were reliable and valid? How would you share that information with your clients?

10. How would you address concerns that were beyond your scope of practice and competence that arose during session? What referral policies and practices would you have in place?

VOICES FROM THE FIELD

Pros and Cons of Career Counseling Remotely

Debra Ruddell, MS, CCC, GCDF

As a career counselors, we wear many "hats," which vary depending on which constituency group or population we serve. Some of these hats may include the Teacher Hat, the Advising Hat, the Helper or Healer Hat, as well as a Strategist Hat. When one is meeting with clients remotely, it is sometimes more difficult to attend to which hat to wear per client needs and whether or not it is a good "fit" for the presenting issues.

Pros

- Allows for more flexible hours to meet with working learners/clients, or nontraditional students
- Multiple platforms to choose from for launching a program
- No commuting or traffic stress
- Possibly fewer distractions

- Fewer interruptions from meetings or staff or colleagues
- May meet with more clients/students in a day or week, than in person

Cons

- No matter which hat is being worn, it is easy to misread verbal or visual cues from our clients via electronic communications
- Clients or students may be easily distracted and less attentive depending on their surroundings; e.g., noise, dogs barking, children playing, another phone ringing, nearby activity, and so forth
- Some clients or students are more technically challenged than others, which makes them more anxious to meet remotely with any counselor
- Must make sure that all platforms are secure and meet ethical guidelines
- Find that my clients are more willing to disclose pertinent information in person
- Sometimes more difficult to make the right first impression
- Sometimes takes longer to build a good working rapport
- Must deal with technical difficulties

In conclusion, when possible I prefer to meet with clients and students in person, which is also a characteristic of my personality; however, when there is no option to do so, I am happy to offer remote options.

CONCLUSION

Career counseling was one of the first professional counseling specializations, and also one of the earliest specializations to adapt technology into its practice. The use of CAGS and CIGS were being used in the 1960s, followed by the transition of massive amounts of career information to online systems via the Occupational Outlook Handbook and the Dictionary of Occupational Titles' transition to the O*Net. As such, delivery of services has been easily adapted to distance modalities. However, services provided may be defined as career planning or career counseling, and these distinctions impact the scope of services and their ethical delivery. The NCDA's ethical codes address the variety of tasks that may be performed including career counseling, career assessment, and providing career information. While DC allows more individuals to access career services, a multitude of challenges exist pertaining to credible information, access, and fees for services. Additionally, social media plays a large role in one's professional image, which may impact an individual's career outcomes. Career counselors need to navigate the inclusion of social media while also maintain professional boundaries. Finally, while global career credentials exist, the lack of state-level licensure for career counselors encourages expansive interactions. While this positively impacts access to services, the lack of state oversight may contribute to unethical or unauthorized services that pose a risk to the public.

REFERENCES

American Counseling Association. (2014). *2014 code of ethics.* https://www.counseling.org/resources/aca-code-of-ethics.pdf

Bright, J. E. H. (2015). If you go down to the woods today you are in for a big surprise: Seeing the wood for the trees in online delivery of career guidance. *British Journal of Guidance & Counselling, 43,* 24–35. https://doi.org/10.1080/03069885.2014.979760

Brown, D. (2016). *Career information, career counseling, and career development* (11th ed.). Pearson.

Harris-Bowlsbey, J., & Sampson. (2005). Use of technology in delivering career services worldwide. *The Career Development Quarterly, 54,* 48–56. https://doi.org/10.1002/j.2161-0045.2005.tb00140.x

Jacobson, M. D., & Grabowski, B. T. (1981). Computerized systems of career information and guidance: A state-of-the-art. *Education Resource Information System (ERIC).* https://files.eric.ed.gov/fulltext/ED210552.pdf

Kettunen, J., Sampson, J. P., & Vuorinen, R. (2015). Career practitioners' conceptions of competency for social media in career services. *British Journal of Guidance & Counseling, 43,* 43–56. https://doi.org/10.1080/03069885.2014.939945

Mulcahy Boer, P. (2009). *Career counseling over the Internet: An emerging model for trusting and responding to online clients.* Lawrence Erlbaum Associates Inc. Publishers.

National Career Development Association. (2015a). *NCDA Code of Ethics.* https://ncda.org/aws/NCDA/asset_manager/get_file/3395

National Career Development Association. (2015b). *The role of career information and technological resources in career planning.* https://www.ncda.org/aws/NCDA/pt/sd/product/2448/_PARENT/layout_products/false

National Employment Counseling Association. (2001). *National Employment Counseling Competencies.* http://www.employmentcounseling.org/national-employment-counseling-competencies.html

Osborn, D. S., Carr, D. L., McClain Riner, M., Sides, R. D., Lumsden, J. A., & Sampson, J. P. (2019). Computer-assisted career assessment. In K. B. Stoltz & S. R. Barclay (Eds.), *A comprehensive guide to career assessment* (7th ed.). National Career Development Association.

Pew Research Group. (12 June, 2019). *Internet and technology; Mobile fact sheet.* https://www.pewInternet.org/fact-sheet/mobile

Sampson, J. P., & Makela, J. P. (2014). Ethical issues associated with information and communication technology in counseling and guidance. *International Journal of Education and Vocational Guidance, 14*, 135–148. http://doi/10.1007/s10775-013-9258-7

United Nations. (2018, December 7). Internet milestone reached, as more than 50 percent go online: UN telecoms agency. *Economic Development.* https://news.un.org/en/story/2018/12/1027991

U.S. Bureau of Labor Statistics. (2019, April 17). *BLS history.* https://www.bls.gov/bls/history/timeline.htm

U.S. Department of Justice, Civil Rights Division. (2003). Web accessibility under Title II of the ADA. *ADA Best Practices Toolkit for State and Local Government.* https://www.ada.gov/pcatoolkit/chap5toolkit.htm

Venable, M. A. (2010). Using technology to deliver career development services: Supporting today's students in higher education. *The Career Development Quarterly, 59*, 87–96.

8

Assessment and Research Using Telemental Health

INTRODUCTION

The Council on the Accreditation of Counseling and Related Education Programs (CACREP) standards are composed of both common core standards and counseling specialty standards. Assessment and Research are two of the common core areas required in the training of master's level counselors (CACREP, 2016). Among the CACREP specialty area standards, assessment or diagnosis is mentioned in Addiction Counseling, Career Counseling, Mental Health Counseling, Clinical Rehabilitation Counseling, College Counseling and Student Affairs, Marriage Couple and Family Counseling, School Counseling, and Rehabilitation Counseling. In fact, every counseling specialization indicates required training in assessment and/or diagnosis beyond the common core area of assessment. Interestingly, none of the CACREP specialty areas in the 2016 standards mention research beyond the core area standards.

All counseling specializations engage in assessment and/or diagnosis for the population they serve, despite misconceptions that these tasks are reserved for mental health practitioners. While CACREP specializations don't specifically mention research beyond the core area, all specialty areas address either program evaluation or data management. Due to the emphasis on assessment, this chapter focuses primarily on assessment via distance counseling (DC) and telemental health (TMH), yet will also address common concerns and guidelines in conducting distance research. The Association of Assessment and Research in Counseling (AARC) is the professional counseling organization devoted to research and assessment.

Neither TMH nor DC is specifically mentioned in the Assessment and Research CACREP standards, yet both standards require students to be trained in "ethical and culturally relevant strategies" for assessment and research (CACREP, 2016, p. 14). TMH has been found to be effective with diverse and hard-to-reach populations, including rural populations, persons with disabilities, veterans, and individuals who don't readily access counseling. As such, delivering assessment and research via distance modalities can be considered a culturally responsive strategy to address these populations. As with DC/TMH counseling services, however, the populations served by distance assessment and research must have the technological, cognitive, developmental, and economic capabilities to access these services.

TELEMENTAL HEALTH ASSESSMENT

The earliest TMH practices included assessment, beginning with the first telemedicine study in 1959 to evaluate patients' psychiatric needs (Breen & Matusitz, 2010). Telepsychiatry was common by the 1990s (American Psychiatric Association [APA], n.d.). Beyond psychiatry, professional counselors have advocated for ethical assessment via the Internet for over two decades. Specifically, counselors have promoted how the Internet plays a role in enhancing the assessment phases of test selection, orientation, administration, scoring and interpretation (Sampson, 2000).

Test Selection

The Internet allows counselors to access a vast amount of information, exploring various test options for the clients and students they serve. Internet research and test repositories permit counselors to identify assessments for multiple populations and clinical issues. Additionally, counselors can research the reliability and validity of each assessment, and link directly to publisher information (Sampson, 2000). Conversely, there are concerns that the Internet provides access to a variety of instruments that may not be valid or reliable, including those without sound psychometric properties. When a valid and reliable paper test is adapted to online delivery, that assessment must then be normed for reliability and validity in the online version (Klion, 2016; Munro Cullum & Gosch, 2013) before it can be used ethically. Digital versions of assessments should be subjected to test-retest reliability from the paper to digital format (Klion, 2016). Because of the ease of putting information on the Internet and creating digital versions of surveys and assessments (Dombeck, 2016), these critical steps may be overlooked. Counselors must select only instruments that are appropriate for the population and clinical issue being served, as well as instruments that are reliable and valid for online administration. Counselors must select assessments that are appropriate for the client's clinical issue and cognitive function, as well as considering any sensory issues that may impact the client's ability to access the selected technology (Luxton et al., 2016).

Test Orientation

Orienting the client, student, or family to the purpose of the assessment facilitates client trust and assists the client, student, or family in understanding the role and function of the assessment. The orientation phase also allows clients and students to ask questions or clarify information that may be unclear. Posting orientation information on a website, digital document, or video can ensure that consistent information is provided to clients, students, and family members on the assessment process. Sampson (2000) points out that the orientation phase may become repetitive to test facilitators, who may miss important aspects of the overview or vary information for some recipients. Technological delivery minimizes those common cause variations, yet also reduces the capacity for clients, students, and family to ask questions or seek clarification from a live counselor. For these reasons, utilizing technology such as telephone or video conferencing would allow test subjects access to a live counselor, if needed.

The orientation phase includes the review of a detailed informed consent document, via which clients and/or family members are made aware of the purpose of the assessment. These DC/TMH informed consent documents must include information on the limits of technology, plans for technology failure, and a detailed safety plan. Similar to other DC/TMH services such as individual and group counseling, informed consents also include a detailed safety plan. Before engaging a client in DC/TMH assessment, the counselor is aware of the laws and statutes in their state which impact TMH assessments. The counselor should also be aware of any limits that insurance companies may have with DC/TMH assessments (Luxton et al., 2016). Counselors address these concerns with clients during the orientation phase, and prior to providing services.

Test Administration

The benefits of administering assessments via the Internet mirror other DC/TMH interventions. These include reducing logistical costs of travel associated with treatment, as well as reaching test subjects in rural areas or those who have limited mobility (Munro Cullum & Gosch, 2013). Online assessment reduces the costs of administration and publishing (Dombeck, 2016). Another benefit of online testing is the ability to receive assessment feedback from multiple perspectives or collateral contacts without having to schedule individual sessions (Klion, 2016). This can be particularly helpful for parent–teacher rating scales or other instruments that require input from multiple sources. Despite these benefits, there are concerns that administering tests online impacts the purity of the test environment, particularly if the client is taking the test in their home or if the test is supposed to be administered in a supervised setting (Klion, 2016). Factors, such as interference from parents, guardians, or others, may influence the subject's performance and results may be impacted by the environment in which the testing occurred.

Technological issues may also impact the test administration, including service disruption, slow connections, and lost data. Administering a test on a computer provides some benefits for displaying images (Sampson, 2000), such as 3D or color images, but may limit test administration that requires the client to use manipulatives (Munro Cullum & Gosch, 2013). Manipulatives are often used in assessments to assess dexterity, or demonstrate interactions with objects. For example, diagnostic vocational evaluation tools, such as the Skills Assessment Module (SAM; Piney Mountain Press, 2008) or the Talent Assessment Program (TAP; Talent Assessment Inc., n.d.), require subjects to manipulate objects, including wiring, tools, and item sorts to measure dexterity, cognitive processing, and spatial relations. Adapting assessments such as these to an online environment would be challenging. As stated, the instrument must have been designed and validated for online use. The American Counseling Association (ACA, 2014) ethical codes remind counselors that assessments must be supervised unless developed for self-administration. This ethical guideline serves to caution counselors who may be tempted to adapt in-person test administration to an unsupervised, online setting.

Scoring and Interpretation

The ease of scoring online assessments and generating assessment reports is often cited as a primary benefit of online assessment. The computer program minimizes the possibility of human error, particularly for repetitive tasks such as scoring assessments (Sampson, 2000). However, by removing the scoring responsibility from the counselor, computer programs focus strictly on the reported outcomes, as opposed to any circumstances or anomalies that a human scorer would have noted via hand scoring. There is a concern that when self-administered assessments are automatically scored, clients lose the opportunity to interpret results with a qualified counselor, particularly with self-help online assessments. Computer-scored results report outcomes based only on numerical data and fail to account for client history or context (Dombeck, 2016).

Counselors have a responsibility to share results once tests are scored. Counselors provide ethical interpretation to clients, students, or family members, or as a consultant. Test results can be shared with clients, students, or parents via DC/TMH modalities including videoconferencing, telephone, and email, with appropriate consent documents and security measures. In order to avoid Health Insurance Portability and Accountability Act (HIPAA) violations or data breaches, subjects may be able to sign in to a secure portal to view their results confidentially. Assessment results may generate treatment recommendations. DC/TMH assessment is used in settings where clients have limited access to clinicians, or when clients cannot readily access clinical services. Regardless of the counselor's location, the counselor should be prepared to assist the client in locating any recommended services that the DC/TMH assessment generates (Luxton et al., 2016).

Other Assessments

CACREP requires that programs provide training to students on "environmental assessments and systematic behavioral observations" (2016, p. 4), which recognizes that assessment practices include more than standardized tests. Other forms of assessment include intake screenings, diagnostic interviews, collateral interviews, observations, and Mental Status Exams (MSEs), and can also be administered via DC/TMH modalities. Intake screenings are regularly conducted via telephone, since many screenings include a questionnaire of symptoms that can be asked and answered verbally. Intake screenings may also be administered via email or digital forms. Diagnostic and collateral interviews are best administered via videoconferencing. Videoconferencing allows the interviewer to observe the behavior, appearance, and spoken word of the client, student, or parent/family. This audio and video observation allows the interviewer to assess speech, cognition, appearance, and family/caregiver interaction. Specifically, the MSE requires the counselor to observe the subject's rate of speech, appearance, and thought content, which require both visual and auditory feedback, which may be best evaluated by videoconferencing (Munro Cullum & Gosch, 2013) if not in person. Other types of assessment are being developed specifically for online administration, including mobile apps and virtual reality tools (Dombeck, 2016).

Ethics of Assessment

Professional counselors adhere to the standards of the ACA Code of Ethics, which specifies ethical guidelines for assessment, regardless of the delivery modality. Specifically, Section E., Evaluation, Assessment, and Interpretation, details ethical practices including instrument selection, administration, scoring, and interpretation. Other key elements of the codes include understanding the purpose of assessment, focusing on client welfare, informed consent, diagnosing mental disorders, and being aware of multicultural and historical contexts of assessment. Of importance is the code's emphasis on competence (E.2.), specifically that counselors who are using technology-assisted instruments must have received training in administering the tool via technology prior to use. This specifies that counselors who use technology assisted assessments must be trained to competently use, administer, and interpret the assessment.

Several major counseling organizations publish guidelines on ethics in assessment and testing. The AARC provides links to assessment statements from organizations specific to multicultural counseling, career counseling, marriage/couple/family counseling, mental health counseling, and substance abuse counseling. These statements from a multitude of professional organizations reinforce that assessment occurs across disciplines, as opposed to strictly in mental health functions. Further, the AARC provides links to position statements, such as the ACA's position on High Stakes Testing or Pre-Employment Testing under the Americans with Disabilities Act (ADA; AARC, 2020).

ETHICS OF ONLINE RESEARCH

Many practicing counselors do not view research as a component of their daily work with clients and students. Some counselors view research as a component of their academic experience, conducted only in labs, or completed strictly by faculty members in academia (Remley & Herlihy, 2016). The extent to which practicing counselors engage in research varies, yet the foundation of all research, including in-person or online research, is ethics. As discussed, the ACA Code of Ethics specifies that the counselor be competent in technology, regardless of its use in their practice. This standard also applies to the practice of research utilizing online or distance technologies, and ensuring technical, ethical, and legal competence on the part of the researcher. This standard includes the practice of research utilizing online or distance technologies.

Research Subjects' Safety

Counselor competence and subject well-being are at the foundation of the ACA (2014) ethical research standards. The ACA codes specify that counselors conduct research methodically, ethically, and in accordance with laws and governing bodies. Counselors protect subjects' safety and well-being, including avoiding harm to subjects' physical, psychological, or social wellness. The responsibility for subject wellness lies with the primary investigator (PI). As in counseling, research subjects are provided with an informed consent, must participate voluntarily, and have their confidentiality and privacy protected throughout the process. Researchers must explain data collection, inform participants of sponsored research, and maintain professional boundaries. Additional guidelines address reporting, publishing, and presentation of research results (ACA, 2014).

Digital Security

Conducting research online or via technology requires adherence to these standards, yet adds an additional layer of responsibility in relation to security, confidentiality, encryption, and sending and storing data. When utilizing or distributing research materials, including distribution of surveys, disseminating results, or publishing, counselors must adhere to all copyright laws and have authorization to distribute or publish related items (Remley & Herlihy, 2016). Similarly, ethical guidelines emphasize properly crediting authors and contributors. This includes not only citing sources properly in publications, but acknowledging the work that all parties contribute to the research or publication. Internet use leaves a "digital footprint" that demonstrates the online activity of an individual. While some of that footprint is hidden to the public eye, other online activity is public, such as blog posts, public discussion boards, and social media activity. Some researchers gather digital footprint data as a form of conducting online research (Hooley & Dodd, 2016).

Benefits and Risks of Online Research

Distance or online research is a convenient way to gather respondents (Hooley & Dodd, 2016). The ease of distributing research surveys via email, listservs, or websites certainly reaches more individuals than having to view a poster on a bulletin board or receiving information about a study from a practitioner. Soliciting a larger number of respondents via the Internet can provide greater depth to quantitative studies and provide a more realistic evaluation of respondent perspectives. Similarly, tools such as email, listservs, and websites can be used to recruit interview candidates for qualitative studies. These interviews can be conducted via DC/TMH technologies, such as videoconferencing or telephone. These sampling procedures are regularly utilized but may not provide the diversity needed to minimize bias or to generalize results to diverse populations. Depending on which online communities or email lists were utilized to solicit respondents, researchers may (intentionally or unintentionally) target only a small demographic of the larger population.

Respondents lose the opportunity to communicate with a live researcher to articulate questions or concerns during online or digital research. This is particularly important with counseling research, which may trigger an emotional response in subjects. Depending on the technology utilized, visual or auditory cues may be lost during the research. It may be difficult to verify the participant's identity if verification is required for the research (Hooley & Dodd, 2016). When recruiting candidates remotely, there is a possibility that respondents may not fit the research subject profile or may be motivated by online incentives to falsely claim they meet the profile. As with online assessment, when subjects complete research surveys or interviews in their own environment, as opposed to a controlled environment, the integrity of the research environment may be compromised.

Many of these concerns are addressed through standard research protocols. Clearly defining the research subject profile, both in the recruitment and informed consent, will improve subjects' understanding of the qualifications required to participate. Similarly, digital surveys can build in screening questions that require respondents to indicate how they fit the research profile. Many online survey design tools provide mechanisms for survey "branching" or "skip logic," which allows survey designers to branch survey items and skip certain questions based on how respondents answer. When a respondent answers an online question indicating that they don't meet the profile, the survey software can skip the respondent to the end of the survey, explain that they do not fit the profile, and thank them for their time. Even if survey software does not have this technology, it helps to include these screening questions, such that the researcher can remove those respondents that don't fit the research profile from the overall data set.

Lack of human contact during the research process can be addressed by providing contact information for the PI, the Institutional Review Board (IRB), or entity overseeing the research. The researcher can be available via phone, email, or video session to respond to any inquiries. Research that may be emotionally triggering, or in other ways risk client well-being, should be clearly stated in the informed consent. Respondents should have the option of exiting the research at any time. It may be prudent to add a closing page on digital surveys or follow up email with information on support services, depending on the nature of the research and the emotional response required from participants. If identity verification is required before beginning the research, researchers can utilize the same strategies utilized in individual DC/TMH verification including use of photo IDs or respondent-selected code words.

Research Resources

Counselors who are engaging in online research can familiarize themselves with resources provided by the AARC. Specifically, the AARC publishes, *Research Resources,* a compilation of scholarly articles pertaining to the ethical and effective practice of research in counseling (AARC, 2012). Other resources include information on the scientist–practitioner model, which provides an overview of engaging in research as a practitioner (AARC, 2009). This resource emphasizes evidence-based practices, outcome research, statistical significance, power and effect size. For the counseling practitioner looking to expand their understanding of publishing research in counseling, the *Journal of Counseling and Development* published a special edition on research and publication in counseling, including articles on quantitative research, statistical power, meta analyses, action research, qualitative research, ethical research, conceptual articles, and international publications (Hunt & Trusty, 2011). Finally, Wester and Borders (2014) specify research competencies in counseling, indicating that competent counselor-researchers will have knowledge, skills, and attributes in the following areas: Informed and Critical Thinking, the Research Process, Ethical and Professional Competence, Breadth and Appreciation, Relational Aspects, and Continuing Education (pp. 452–455). While not specifically designed for online and distance research, these competencies serve as a measure of competence for all counselors engaging in research.

RESEARCH AND ASSESSMENT DATA

Assessment and research generate data. Both assessment and research involve the collection and storage of client and participant data. As discussed, ethical codes require the use of encryption technology for digital practices, as well as safeguards to protect client information (ACA, 2014). Use of technology introduces risks in data retrieval, data portability, data loss, and connection failures (Klion, 2016). Counselors engaging in online research and assessment are competent to use the required technology, as well as access technological support in the event of system errors.

Technical support should be evaluated by counselors considering online assessment and research technology. Security measures must be put in place in order to protect the privacy of data collected. Transmission of data can utilize encrypted and password-protected systems in order to avoid unauthorized access to individual data. Data must be stored on secure, password protected devices. When using third-party vendors, such as survey creation tools or online test administration software, the security of client data may be at risk. Counselors review third-party vendor privacy policies for information on data access, storage, retrieval, and disposal. For data stored on remote servers or systems, counselors may also need to review the privacy policies of cloud storage systems.

Counselors adhere to data storage and disposal policies within their organization, which includes policies for both digital data and paper data. Digital data must be stored and disposed of properly. Informed consents to participate in research or assessment must include how long and where data will be stored. Finally, counselors inform test subjects and research subjects about the potential loss of data and/or data breeches that may occur with any technological storage and transmission of test and research data. This information is provided in an informed consent, which notifies participants prior to engaging in research or testing, and respects their autonomy to withdraw from the activity.

There has been discussion and debate about data collected from digital footprints or data mining. Data mining is defined as "the process of digging through data to discover hidden connections and predict future trends" (SAS, 2020, para. 2). When counselors use public data to conduct research, it has been argued that human subject rules don't apply to publicly posted data because the researcher is analyzing data as opposed to people (Thelwall, 2010). There are concerns that an individual's online self may not represent their true self, as people regularly portray themselves differently in online spaces. There are questions surrounding the ethics of mining data from public or online communities. While many of these online communities are indeed public, there is a belief that the individuals who post information there intend that information for only a small audience, and not to be utilized for analysis or generalizations to larger audiences (Hooley & Dodd, 2016).

CHALLENGES AND OPPORTUNITIES

Administering assessments and conducting research online or via distance technologies continue to provide both challenges and opportunities for counselors and counseling researchers. As discussed, there are both benefits and risk to online administration of assessments and research. While many of these have been previously addressed, the following items should also be weighed by the counselor considering assessment and/or research via distance technology.

Self-Help Tests

The number of online, self-administered, self-help tests has continued to grow along with the expansion of the Internet. There are multiple concerns about the fact that these self-help assessments are readily available to the public via Internet search engines. Primary concerns are that some instruments are not valid or reliable, have no clinical value, or that they are used to gather market-driven data (Dombeck, 2016). Self-administered and self-scored assessments lack the interpretation and support of a qualified professional counselor to review the results.

Valid and reliable self-help assessments provide benefits to the public, such as making assessments available to a wider audience. There are many well-established, valid, and reliable online self-help assessments, such as the Self-Directed-Search (PAR, 2020) for career counseling or the Veterans Administration's (VA) screening tools for posttraumatic stress disorder (PTSD), depression, substance abuse, and alcohol use (VA, n.d.). In addition, some online assessments can be accessed with a prescription or code from a professional counselor who can then provide support to review assessment results with the client. Self-monitoring tools also provide benefits to clients in order to record daily activity such as emotions, thoughts, or behaviors (Dombeck, 2016).

Lack of Counselor Contact

As discussed, online administration of assessments and research lacks a human connection for questions and concerns, as well as human observation of behavior and distress. Selected technology may impact a counselor's observation and assessment. While MSEs are said to be effective via videoconferencing (Munro Cullum & Gosch, 2013), counselors lose subtle cues of functioning, such as olfactory senses which may be an indication of client wellness. Even among assessments that are designed to be self-administered and self-scored, clients may have uncertainty about their results which require clarification from a professional counselor.

Mobile Apps

The future, if not the present, of research and assessment lies in mobile applications. It is believed that mobile apps will be used to screen candidates for research, and that tests will be designed specifically for mobile app administration. While some argue that small screen size and reduced audio may impact this development (Munro Cullum & Gosch, 2013), online survey creation tools provide multiple view options including views for computers, tablets, and phones. As discussed, the ability for subjects to enter data into a device in real time, either as symptoms occur or via alarm reminders, can provide longitudinal data for issues usually examined in a one-time sitting. The benefit is that these apps allow the client to record symptoms as they occur, as opposed to waiting until a live session, during which the client attempts to recall the onset, frequency, antecedents, intensity, and duration of their symptoms. As with other technology, the security and validity of apps will continue to be a challenge, and users need to be notified of these risks prior to use.

Data Use and Distribution

The Crisis Text Line, launched in 2013, has received over 140 million text messages as a text resource for individuals in crisis (Crisis Text Line, 2020). Its founder, Nancy Lubin, proudly discusses the Crisis Text Line's use of data, both for internal and external support. Internally, data in text messages are used to triage texters to high priority cues, provide suggested text responses, and monitor crisis spikes, surrounding topics, issues, or geographic locations. Externally, the Crisis Text Line shares a great deal of its data publicly, either via its website, published research, or other mechanisms (Crisis Text Line, 2020). For the most part, the public response to data sharing has been positive, yet some groups have questioned the decision to share data while simultaneously protecting texter confidentiality (Hullinger, 2016; Pisani et al., 2019). External data from individuals in crisis are redacted for confidentiality and privacy before distribution. There is also a privacy policy that texters agree to when contacting the hotline; however, the emotional state of the person utilizing the hotline may impact their understanding of those terms. The Crisis Text Line is just one example of the ways in which data mining can be utilized in research. Other examples can be derived from any resource or service that collects individual data to provide a service, and then later utilizes that data to conduct research. Similar discussions have included social media posts, discussion board posts, and blog posts. The information gleaned from these data mining activities can be vast and valuable, yet counseling researchers need to balance those benefits with their perceptions of client privacy.

Data mining is also practiced by unauthorized individuals and entities, and may create opportunities for security breaches or HIIPAA violations. Sobelman and Santopietro (2018) warn that data mining is big business, and that data brokers trade and purchase data via trillions of transactions a day. To prevent unauthorized access to data, they recommend using non-internet based connections when possible, opting out of all data brokering and direct marketing activities, and using data browsers that block cookies. Cookies is a term for a set of data that is sent to one's computer after one visits a website, which is then stored on the computer. The data set contains information which may include personal information pertaining to the website visit (NortonLifeLock, 2020).

CASE STUDY: ASSESSMENT

Counselor A is a mental health provider who is contracted to serve several large school districts in a rural part of the state. Because of the low socioeconomic status of the region, there are no mental health providers employed by the school district. All mental health services are contracted on an as-needed basis to external licensed providers. Client B is a 14-year-old, eighth-grade student who recently was referred to Counselor A for a psychological evaluation and safety assessment. School administrators became concerned about Client B after other students reported that Client B's drawings and writings were "scary." Upon confiscation and viewing the student's writings and drawings, Client B was placed on a medical leave from the school and referred for evaluation. Counselor A's evaluation and assessment is needed for Client B to return to school, and to determine if counseling or hospitalization is necessary, prior to returning.

Client B lives approximately 90 miles from Counselor A. For any client that is more than a 30-minute drive from the office, Counselor A offers TMH appointments. Counselor A also offers TMH for clients without access to transportation since public transit is unavailable in their rural area. Counselor A spoke to Client B's parent in order to arrange the TMH evaluation appointment, and reviewed a detailed informed consent for the TMH session. Client B's parent appeared frustrated by the requirement, stating that the school was "overreacting," and that Client B is simply "creative, artistic, dark, and dramatic." Client B's parent also shared that they believe the referral to administration is another example of how other students "pick on Client B—ever since we moved here in elementary school, the other kids always pick on Client B."

Counselor B planned to administer the Beck Depression Inventory II (BDI; Beck et al., 1996) and the Suicide Assessment Five-Step Evaluation and Triage (SAFE-T; Jacobs, 2009), in addition to a diagnostic interview. Counselor A planned to deliver the SAFE-T assessment via client interview during the video conference. For the BDI, the publisher's website recommends utilizing their proprietary software for administration and scoring during TMH sessions. Counselor A did not purchase the online administration of the BDI, but scanned a paper version, and emailed it to the parent. Counselor A told the parent to have Client B complete the BDI and return the results via email prior to the evaluation meeting.

On the day of the evaluation, Client B appeared on time for the video-conference, along with the parent. Client B was dressed in what appeared to be pajamas, with unkempt hair, slouched posture, and limited eye contact. During the initial introductions and explanations, Client B's parent would often answer on behalf of the child, and provide unsolicited information, such as, "I told Client B to get up earlier to be ready for this meeting. I asked Client B to wear something nicer." Counselor A explained that it would be best if Client B was allowed to answer questions on their own, and that the parent was welcome to leave the room for a period of time so Counselor A and Client B could talk. The parent stated that they prefer to stay in the room but could give Client B some privacy by moving to another part of the room.

DISCUSSION QUESTIONS

1. Think about Counselor A's policies for TMH sessions and preparation for this session. What are some elements of this case that might require special attention if using TMH?

2. Discuss Counselor A's use of assessments, including her plan to conduct a diagnostic interview, as well as use the BDI and SAFE-T. How did using TMH impact these decisions? What concerns do you have about the use of assessments in this case, if any?

3. How would you have managed the behavior of Client B's parent during the session? In what ways was having the parent there helpful? In what ways was it harmful?

4. Discuss Counselor A's ability to build rapport with Client B. How did the TMH support or hinder that relationship?

5. Assuming good intent, what did Counselor A do well?

CRITICAL QUESTIONS IN DECIDING TO PRACTICE

Counselors who conduct assessment and research in traditional, face-to-face settings, may be considering a transition to online or distance modalities. Similarly, counselors may already be conducting research and assessment in online or distance formats, but have not reflected previously on the process. The reflection questions that follow are designed to help counselors assess their competence and comfort in administering online assessments and research.

1. What training and experience do you currently have in assessment? What type of assessments have you administered previously and in what format? How much of your training involves administering these instruments online?

2. What do you know about the assessments you currently administer and their use in online settings? Were these assessments normed and validated for online use? What are the publishers' recommendations pertaining to online administration?

3. If you were to administer online or distance assessment, what adaptations to your current practice would you need to make? How would you facilitate test selection, orientation, administration, and interpretation in an online setting, as opposed to an in-person setting?

4. What type of training and experience do you have in research? How would you evaluate your competence in relation to Wester and Borders (2014) research competencies?

5. How do you feel about online research, including elements such as recruiting respondents via online modalities, conducting research via online modalities, and data mining? Which of these practices concern you, if at all? Why?

6. If you were to engage in online research what adaptations to your research practices would you need to make, if any? What modalities would you use?

7. Consider the technology you would use for either online research or assessment. What steps would you need to take to ensure that the technology you use is secure and encrypted? How would you determine the appropriate technological intervention/tool?

8. How would you overcome the absence of human presence in the testing or research environment? How might the absence of the counselor impact your assessment or research results, if at all?

9. How would you store the data from your assessment and research? What policies do you need to follow for safe data storage, transmission, and disposal? Would you be required to review any third-party privacy policies?

10. What ethical issues impact your practice? How would you safeguard client well-being, while also protecting the integrity of the results? How would you articulate the risks of online research or assessment to the clients or respondents who participate?

VOICES FROM THE FIELD

Determining a Diagnosis Using Telemental Health

Christopher E. Fisher, PsyD, MSEd

In March of 2020, I began working in a group private practice with hopes of diversifying my clinical experience from my full-time position as an inpatient clinical psychologist at a large local community hospital. However, beginning outpatient work at the outbreak of the COVID-19 pandemic triggered more uncertainty and ambiguity than is considered typical of the therapeutic process, both for my clients and myself. The daily media updates on the increasing number of total cases and death rates in the United States via COVID-19 has not only exacerbated fear and panic in existing clients, but it has also sparked uneasiness and discomfort among individuals not currently engaged in treatment. Additionally, mandated stay-at-home and social distancing orders significantly changed the frame under which my treatment took place. In attempts to accommodate these unprecedented times of uncertainty, the decision was made to transition to telemental health (TMH) counseling. This transition has been quite the adjustment as it brings about an abundance of pros, but also encompasses various cons.

Limited by the orders already mentioned TMH counseling has allowed access to mental health care during a time of great need. TMH counseling has provided a sense of connectedness, support, and safety for those seeking help to effectively cope with their daily struggles of unpleasant feelings and thoughts associated with the COVID-19 pandemic. Despite these pros, aspects of my responsibility as a mental health clinician have become increasingly more challenging during this transition, particularly rapport building and assigning accurate diagnoses. Throughout my years of training and practice, I have utilized face-to-face interaction as my primary therapeutic frame of delivering treatment. I believe this particular method of carrying out treatment has always provided me the support necessary to build a strong and essential foundational therapeutic relationship with my clients. Due to the highly contractible nature of COVID-19 and efforts to maintain social distancing orders, my ability to provide face to face treatment has been suppressed. This has left me with many questions and concerns as I entered into uncharted territory. Given this new sense of uncertainty, it was as if my own unfamiliarity with TMH counseling began to mirror the experience of my clients who were also new to this type of treatment delivery.

During my initial psychodiagnostic evaluations with new clients, I perform semi-structured clinical interviews intended to gather both the present and historical information needed to determine an appropriate diagnosis and establish goals to guide the treatment process. My inability to trust my capability to engage clients in this new context affected my confidence level in not only making accurate diagnoses, but also instilling hope in clients questioning whether this form of treatment was worth it, whether it would be beneficial. My intake evaluations have been bombarded with more time focused fielding questions regarding the context of treatment and trying to "hook" my clients into continuing with treatment, meaning less time was focused on gathering the necessary information for diagnostic clarity. "You never want to make a diagnosis in the first session" was something that was preached during my years of graduate school. This concept was quickly challenged when entering into a world governed by insurance reimbursements. The inner conflict I felt between assigning an accurate diagnosis and providing a preliminary diagnosis for billing purposes is one that has been hard to hold.

Advice I would share for clinicians transitioning into TMH counseling would be for them to remain adaptable, and provide as much information as possible prior to treatment beginning with the context of TMH counseling itself with new clients. This might include, but not be limited to, forms of accepted payment, cancellation and rescheduling policies, and technological malfunctions and troubleshooting.

CONCLUSION

Technology can be utilized to enhance both assessment and research procedures, yet counselors engaging in these practices must also exercise caution. Test selection is improved through expansive resources, yet selected assessments must be appropriate for distance administration. Selected assessments must be normed and validated in an online environment. Test orientation, administration, and scoring/interpretation is also enhanced by the speed and accessibility that technology provides; however, there are concerns that the integrity of the testing environment may be compromised by technology slowdowns or interruptions. In addition, loss of some sensory cues, such as sight, sound, or olfactory senses, may impact the outcome of assessments, such as mental status exams. Online research has the ability to capture data from a wide range of participants, but the researcher has a responsibility to protect subjects' safety while also maintaining digital security. In both assessment and research, the ability to reach more subjects, minimize travel costs, and provide services to those in need are benefits of the practice. Conversely, the distance administration of these tasks may sacrifice human connection and integrity of the testing/research environments. Counselors engaging in distance research and assessment must ensure ethical storage, retrieval and transmission of client and subject data.

REFERENCES

American Counseling Association. (2014). *2014 ACA code of ethics.* https://www .counseling.org/Resources/aca-code-of-ethics.pdf

American Psychiatric Association. (n.d.). *Telepsychiatry tool kit: History of telepsychiatry.* https://www.psychiatry.org/psychiatrists/practice/telepsychia try/toolkit/history-of-telepsychiatry

Association of Assessment and Research in Counseling. (2009). *The scientist practitioner model: The ethical choice.* https://kxo.052.myftpupload.com/ wp-content/uploads/2020/01/practitioner.pdf

Association of Assessment and Research in Counseling. (2012). *Association for Assessment in Counseling and Education (AACE) research resources.* https://kxo.052. myftpupload.com/wp-content/uploads/2020/01/Research_Resource_List.pdf

Association of Assessment and Research in Counseling. (2020). *Resources.* http:// aarc-counseling.org/resources

Beck, A. T., Steer, R. A., & Brown, G. K. (1996). *Beck Depression Inventory-II.* Pearson. https://www.pearsonassessments.com/store/usassessments/en/ Store/Professional-Assessments/Personality-%26-Biopsychosocial/Beck -Depression-Inventory-II/p/100000159.html

Breen, G. M., & Matusitz, J. (2010). An evolutionary examination of telemedicine: A health and computer-mediated communication perspective. *Social Work Public Health, 25*(1), 59–71. https://doi.org/10.1080/19371910902911206

Council on the Accreditation of Counseling and Related Education Programs. (2016). *2016 CACREP Standards and Glossary.* http://www.cacrep.org/wp -content/uploads/2018/05/2016-Standards-with-Glossary-5.3.2018.pdf

Crisis Text Line. (2020). *Data philosophy.* https://www.crisistextline.org/ data-philosophy

Dombeck, M. (2016). Use of online psychological testing for self-help. In S. Goss, K. Anthony, L. Sykes Stretch, & D. Merz Nagel (Eds.), *Technology in mental health: Applications in practice, supervision, and training.* Charles C. Thomas Publishers.

Hooley, T., & Dodd, V. (2016). Online research methods for mental health. In S. Goss, K. Anthony, L. Sykes Stretch, & D. Merz Nagel (Eds.), *Technology in mental health: Applications in practice, supervision, and training.* Charles C. Thomas Publishers.

Hullinger, J. (2016, February 22). Crisis text line is opening a treasure trove of data to researchers. *Fast Company.* https://www.fastcompany.com/3056936/ crisis-text-line-is-opening-its-treasure-trove-of-data-to-researchers

Hunt, B., & Trusty, J. (2011). Counseling research and publishing in JCD: Introduction to the special section. *Journal of Counseling & Development, 89,* 256–260. https://doi.org/10.1002/j.1556-6678.2011.tb00086.x

Jacobs, D. (2009). *Suicide Assessment Five-Step Evaluation and Triage (SAFE-T).* https://www.integration.samhsa.gov/images/res/SAFE_T.pdf

Klion, R. E. (2016). Web based clinical assessment. In S. Goss, K. Anthony, L. Sykes Stretch, & D. Merz Nagel (Eds.), *Technology in mental health: Applications in practice, supervision, and training.* Charles C. Thomas Publishers.

Luxton, D. D., Nelson, E., & Maheu, M. M. (2016). *A practitioner's guide to telemental health: How to conduct legal, ethical, and evidence-based telepractice.* American Psychological Association.

Munro Cullum, C., & Gosch, M. C. (2013). Special considerations in conducting neuropsychology assessment over videoteleconferencing. In K. Myers & C. Turvey (Eds.), *Telemental health: Clinical, technical, and administrative foundations for evidence-based practice.* Elsevier.

NortonLifeLock. (2020). *What are cookies?* https://us.norton.com/internetsecurity-how-to-what-are-cookies.html

PAR. (2020). *Self-Directed Search.* http://www.self-directed-search.com

Piney Mountain Press. (2008). *Skills Assessment Module.* http://www.piney mountain.com/cart/pages/sam.html

Pisani, A. R., Kanuri, N., Filbin, B., Gallo, C., Gould, M., Soleymani Lehmann, L., Levine, R., Marcotte, J. E., Pascal, B., Rousseau, D., Turner, S., Yen, S., & Ranney, M. L. (2019). Protecting user privacy and rights in academic data-sharing partnerships: Principles from a pilot program at Crisis Text Line. *Journal of Medical Internet Research, 21*(1), e11507. https://doi.org/10.2196/11507

Remley, Jr., T. P., & Herlihy, B. (2016). *Ethical, legal, and professional issues in counseling.* Pearson.

Sampson, Jr., J. P. (2000). Using the Internet to enhance testing in counseling. *Journal of Counseling and Development, 78,* 348–356. https://doi.org/10.1002/j.1556-6676.2000.tb01917.x

SAS. (2020). *Data mining: What it is and why it matters?* https://www.sas.com/en_us/insights/analytics/data-mining.html

Sobelman, S. A., & Santopietro, J. M. (2018). Managing risk: Aligning technology use with the law, ethics codes, and practice standards. In J. J. Magnavita (Ed.), *Using technology in mental health practice.* American Psychological Association.

Talent Assessment Inc. (n.d.). *TAP – Functional work skills assessment.* http://www.talentassessment.com/TAP.html

Thelwall, M. (2010, July 12). *Researching the public web.* https://www.ehumanities.nl/researching-the-public-web

Veterans Administration. (n.d.). *Mental health screening tools.* https://www.myhealth.va.gov/mhv-portal-web/screening-tools

Wester, K. L., & Borders, L. D. (2014). Research competencies in counseling: A Delphi study. *Journal of Counseling and Development, 92,* 447–458. https://doi.org/10.1002/j.1556-6676.2014.00171.x

9

Specialized Areas of Practice: Children, Adolescents, and College Students via Telemental Health

INTRODUCTION

The use of distance counseling (DC) and telemental health (TMH) counseling expanded exponentially during the COVID-19 crisis. On March 13, 2020, President Trump declared a national emergency in the United States due to the COVID-19 pandemic, and by March 30, 256 million Americans were required to stay home. These orders impacted students, teachers, and counselors working in classroom K-12 schools and colleges across the country, including the nation's largest school district, New York City, which educates 1.1 million students per day (Taylor, 2020). While campuses and schools were closed, education continued via remote and online instruction, requiring school counselors and student affairs counselors to quickly transition to DC practices. While these transitions were abrupt and unfamiliar to many counselors, online services for K-12 and college student are not new. Universities have utilized online instruction and distance learning practices for decades, including distance support services for students. More recently, online learning for K-12 students has emerged to support students who are home-schooled or home-bound. DC has been successfully utilized with children, adolescents, and young adults in a variety of clinical studies and practical applications. Like all DC/TMH services, counselors providing DC/TMH in K-12 and college settings must be trained in DC delivery and use secure and encrypted technology. They must review a detailed informed consent document with clients/students/parents outlining technology risks and benefits that includes a detailed safety plan or emergency contact plan. As always, counselors must be competent to use technology for DC/TMH interventions, and must assess the competence, preference, access, and ability of the client or student before using distance interventions.

SCHOOL COUNSELING

Today's children and adolescents would likely be described as digital natives (Prensky, 2001), indicating that, for the entirety of their lives, technology has been woven in to the fabric of society. Today's children and adolescents are more connected now than ever. Just over half of all children in the United States (53%) have a smartphone by age 11, and the number increases to 84% by the time they are teenagers (Kamenetz, 2019). Students report that they use their phones primarily to pass time, connect with others, and learn information. To a lesser extent, students report being on their phone to avoid interacting with others (Schaeffer, 2019). These statistics indicate that children and adolescents may be more likely to acclimate to DC services based on their current technology use. While not focused specifically on mobile phone interactions, research demonstrates effective DC/TMH interactions with children and adolescents. In addition, the American School Counselors Association (ASCA) provides essential ethical guidelines to shape the school counselor's role in providing DC to the students they serve.

Effectiveness With Children/Adolescents

Psychiatrists, psychologists, and mental health providers have effectively utilized TMH to address a variety of child and adolescent issues including attention-deficit hyperactive disorder (ADHD), medication management, disruptive behavior disorders, obsessive compulsive disorder (OCD), and parent–child training programs (Comer et al., 2017; McCarty et al., 2015).

The use of TMH can help address the shortage of child and adolescent psychiatrists (Pullen et al., 2013), and has produced outcomes not inferior to those receiving face-to-face (F2F) services. Meta-analyses have revealed positive outcomes for children and adolescents receiving computer-based cognitive behavioral therapy (CBT) for issues of anxiety and depression (Pennant et al., 2015). TMH services can be provided in children's and adolescents' homes, yet can also be provided in school settings. Receiving TMH services in schools may be more convenient for parents and students, and also reduce stigma with receiving mental health care (Stephan et al., 2016). While school-based TMH services are effective, it is recommended that schools have the technological infrastructure to manage TMH services, and that a counselor is on site when TMH services are being conducted. It is also recommended that TMH services not interfere with class schedules, and that providers follow school policies, such as permissions, confidentiality, and special education guidelines (Stephan et al., 2016). Providers who have more training in technology are more likely to utilize TMH services effectively and confidently with children and adolescents (Carlson et al., 2006; Pullen et al., 2013; Steele et al., 2015).

Ethical Codes

This book utilizes the term "distance counseling" in addition to TMH, because school counselors may not resonate with the term "telemental health" counseling. This is because school counselors focus on students' academic, career, and personal/social/emotional concerns per the ASCA Model. The ASCA Ethical Standards for School Counselors (2016) recognizes, however, that school counselors are actively engaging in virtual and DC. Before addressing distance and virtual counseling, the ASCA standards focus on critical elements such as obtaining informed consent, obtaining minor assent, and protecting confidentiality, student safety, and well-being. These are foundational elements of school counseling practice that cannot be overlooked when practicing virtually.

The ASCA Ethical Standards (2016) address technology at multiple points beyond their standalone sections on DC. Beginning with confidentiality, section A.2.k. requires school counselors to recognize the "vulnerability of confidentiality in electronic communications" (p. 2), and requires that they only send information via formats that follow state, federal, and school policies. Additionally, standard A.2.o. recognizes that certain software systems present a risk to student confidentiality, and counselors are advised to "avoid using software programs without the technological capabilities to protect student information" (p. 2). In addressing dual relationships and boundaries, the ASCA standard A.5.d. cautions school counselors about the use of personal accounts to interact with students and parents, specifically stating "do not use personal social media, personal email accounts or personal texts to interact with students unless specifically encouraged and sanctioned by the school district" (p. 3). Regarding student records, standard A.12.e. cautions that electronic communications must comply with the Federal Education Rights and Privacy Act (FERPA) as well as state laws. These precautionary standards remind counselors that—even when not operating in a distance or virtual capacity—technology can create obstacles for ethical practice, simply by using communication systems, software systems, and social media.

The ASCA standards have two standalone sections dedicated to distance and virtual services. Section A.14 Technical and Digital Citizenship reminds school counselors to use technology to enhance students' academic, career, and social/emotional development, while also being mindful of confidentiality and security concerns. This section also requires counselors to maintain confidentiality of student records, promote safe technology use, explain the benefits and limitations of technology, use approved means for communication, and maintain boundaries. This standard requires that school counselors "advocate for equal access to technology for all students" (p. 6). Section A.15 Virtual/Distance School Counseling begins by requiring school counselors to adhere to the same ethical standards and guidelines during DC services as when providing F2F services. It requires school counselors to inform students and parents/families of the benefits and risks of DC, including risks to confidentiality and misinterpretation of nonverbal cues that impact the counseling relationship. Importantly, this section requires school counselors to "implement procedures for students to follow in both emergency and nonemergency situations when the school counselor is not available" (p. 6).

A final important reminder concerns FERPA. It is the school's responsibility to protect students' academic records, and to ensure that information is not distributed to any unauthorized individual. Thus when providing DC services, school counselors must ensure that proper protections and encryption methods are in place to properly safeguard student information. Similarly, school counselors must comply with all state, federal, and local laws to protect student information from security breaches and unauthorized access.

Accessibility

Technology is not evenly distributed. As has been discussed, there are great disparities among those who have access to technology and those who do not. Technology, specifically Internet and broadband access, is more accessible to individuals who are White college-graduates with incomes over $70,000 per year and live in suburban areas (Pew Research Group, 2019). These technological inequalities were made abundantly clear during the COVID-19 crisis when schools moved to distance learning platforms almost overnight. While some districts utilized digital learning and videoconferencing software, others scrambled to distribute loaner laptops or printed paper packages of materials. These disparities were recognized in school districts less than 30 miles apart but with tremendous socioeconomic differences—areas such as Arlington, Virginia, Washington DC, and Prince George's County, Maryland (Troung, 2020). Certain cultural groups, such as Native populations (Groetzinger, 2020) or those in rural areas (Siegler, 2020), also struggle to gain Internet access. Some students are only able to access the Internet via mobile phones.

These concepts are critical considerations for school counselors and school districts using and/or requiring technology in their programs, including DC. Children and adolescents are born into unequal and unjust circumstances, often with limited power and opportunity to advocate for themselves. As such, the ASCA standards specify that school counselors' Responsibilities to the School (B.2) include advocating for equitable school counseling programs, translators for multilingual services, learning needs of all students, cultural competence, equity, and access for all students.

School Counselors' Role

School counselors have been using technology to complete their daily functions for decades. Studies that were conducted nearly two decades ago revealed that 92% of school counselors surveyed were comfortable with computers and 96% were using email. Not surprisingly, however, school counselors who had more training expressed greater comfort (Carlson et al., 2006) and used technology more (Steele et al., 2015). Those numbers have likely maintained or increased since that time. Despite their comfort with computers and email, Wilczenski and Coomey (2006) noted that there were no fully online Council on the Accreditation of Counseling and Related Education Programs (CACREP) school counseling programs at that time (2006), and questions arose as to how school counseling could be taught in an online format. Fast forward to 2020, however, and there are over 20 fully online CACREP accredited school counseling programs (CACREP, 2020). Counselors are not only learning school counseling online but practicing via distance modalities as well. In a pre-COVID-19 study of 771 school counselors' use of technology, approximately 50% of school counselors stated that they used technology for consultation and collaboration, 28%

for classroom guidance, and 26% for group and individual counseling (Steele et al., 2015). When using technology, school counselors made efforts to protect student confidentiality. School counselors expressed challenges with work/home boundaries, as 67% of respondents indicated that they responded to nonurgent student messages outside of working hours. Counselors expressed concerns about helping students in crisis via DC, although 62% reported that they have never received a crisis message from a student outside of working hours (Steele et al., 2015).

School counselors may perform some or all of their functions via DC or virtual counseling. While several school counselors transitioned to distance services during the COVID-19 pandemic, other school counselors serve students enrolled in virtual schools, including students who are home schooled, as well as those enrolled in public and private schools (Osborn et al., 2015). Interviews with virtual school counselors reveal these counselors have a desire to be on the cutting edge of technology and receive increased training in technology multiple times per year. Counselors at a virtual school in the state of Florida have ratios of almost 3,000 to one, and report regularly working beyond traditional school day hours. These counselors explain how they have detailed emergency plans for students in crisis, those expressing suicidality, and in reporting abuse and neglect, although the majority of their student contacts involve academic advising. Virtual school counselors use multiple modalities including phone, email, and videoconferencing, and productivity is monitored via a ticket tracking system which monitors contacts made throughout the day. Described as "early adapters and pioneers" (p. 187) in the virtual school counseling realm, those interviewed expressed the benefits of not having administrative school roles (e.g., bus duty), but also expressed concerns about being able to make accommodations for students with special needs, having to advocate for a student within their home school district, as well as multicultural issues (Osborn et al., 2015).

Social media may also be a concern for school counselors. While the ASCA standards provide guidelines for counselors on their own social media, as well as guidance to instruct students on responsible digital citizenship, social media continues to be a focal point for many adolescents. Whether practicing F2F or virtually, school counselors are likely to have adolescents bring up concerns pertaining to social media. School counselors are encouraged to adapt their communication and thinking surrounding social media to understand the importance of social media to adolescents. Interviews with school counselors found that there was a digital divide between school counselor's connection to the importance of social media for adolescents. These same interviews revealed both fear and frustration among school counselors regarding their students' social media use, but also a need to embrace the emergence of social media and to be prepared to address it in counseling (Gallo et al., 2016–2017). It is recommended that school counselors consider classroom guidance lessons around social media, digital footprints, and Internet dangers, as well as be prepared to provide webinars or other information to parents on these topics (Gallo et al., 2016–2017).

Classroom guidance lessons are a component of many school counselor roles. The transition to distance classroom guidance lessons has benefits as reported in previous literature and research on distance education. Specifically, the National Research Center on Distance Education and Technology Advancements (DETA) publishes eight quality indicators for online classes (Joosten et al., 2019). Specifically, quality online instruction includes: (a) online classes with measurable objectives, (b) classes that are well organized and easy to navigate, (c) support services to students, (d) clarity and reduced barriers to learning, (e) instructor interaction, (f) peer interaction, (g) student interaction with the content of their learning, and (h) rich and varied learning sources to support students' different learning styles (Joosten et al., 2019). In addition, the International Society for Technology (ISTE, 2020) provides standards for students, educators, and school leaders on the integration of technology into the learning environment. School counselors can utilize these professional resources, as well as others, to enhance their classroom guidance materials in their transition to distance counseling. ASCA (2020) provided a variety of free resources on DC to the public in response to the COVID-19 crisis. In addition to materials and lessons for school counselors, they provide virtual toolkits on DC for elementary, middle, and high school counselors with multiple lessons for various grade levels.

Other recommendations for distance school counselors reflect elements outlined in the ASCA Standards. School counselors are encouraged to limit communications and response times. They are encouraged to inform parents and students in advance of these limitations, as well as the risks and benefits of online communication (Steele et al., 2015). School counselors should be prepared for inquiries from parents about social media, limits to social media, and if/how social media seeps into the school setting (Gallo et al., 2016–2017). Finally, school counselors providing distance services need to provide detailed informed consent documents, and have specified emergency procedures in the event of crises or the need to report abuse/neglect (Osborn et al., 2015). Before embarking on any distance or virtual counseling practice, school counselors must check with their school district and state boards to determine any policies and procedures pertaining to virtual services. A school counselor should not operate independently of their districts policies and protocols. All services provided virtually need to be offered equitably and without bias. School policies should specify which services a school counselor is able to offer virtually and under what circumstances. Publicly posted policies, along with any required consent forms, will minimize discrepancies in service delivery.

CASE STUDY: SCHOOL COUNSELING

Counselor A is a school counselor in an urban high school with a population of students from low socioeconomic families. Because of the COVID-19 school closures, Counselor A decides to adapt the traditional classroom guidance lesson on the college search process to a virtual counseling format. Counselor A had adapted the individual sessions and parent consultations to DC, but had not previously conducted a classroom guidance lesson via DC. This classroom guidance lesson is traditionally taught to high school juniors during their English class, which normally has approximately 24 students in a class. In order to make the lessons more personalized, Counselor A is offering the lesson three times for each class, in order to keep the counseling groups capped at eight students in a session. Counselor A will need to conduct the lesson 12 times in order to accommodate all juniors during their English class. To prepare for the lesson, Counselor A emails the first group of students a link to a secure videoconference meeting, a PowerPoint, and informs students that a parent or guardian may wish to attend the group along with the student.

The first classroom guidance session begins and Counselor A notices that there are 15 participants in the group. Out of the eight invited students, five elected to have a parent join who signed in to the classroom from a different device/location than their student. In addition, two students had been forwarded the email from classmates in the group and mistakenly assumed that they were supposed to attend. Counselor A allowed those students to stay in the class. Counselor A explained that they would be recording the class for students and parents to view at a later time. Several students verbally complained about not wanting to be recorded. Counselor A shared the screen with a PowerPoint. After spending about 10 minutes taking attendance and being sure that everyone knew how to use the technology, Counselor A spent about 30 minutes discussing various elements of the college search process. Throughout the process, there was a lot of background noise and students continually yelled at one another to mute themselves. At some point before Counselor A finished the presentation, four members left the group. Counselor A asked if there were any questions at the end of group. There were none and the meeting ended.

For the second group meeting, Counselor A emailed the second group of students a link to a secure videoconference meeting, a Power-Point, and informed them that they cannot have a parent join the meeting, but that the class would be recorded for parents to view at a later date. They also explained that the video would be emailed to parents and not posted publicly. When the second video session starts, Counselor A only has four of the eight students signed in to the class. Counselor A waits 10 minutes for other students to join, and also asks students to reach out to their peers to see if they are having difficulty logging on. One student explained, "They're not coming. They are just going to watch the video later." Another student added, "Plus their mom said they aren't allowed to be recorded, so they didn't have to attend." Before the meeting starts, Counselor A tells all students to put their microphones on mute and wait until the end of the lesson to ask any questions. Counselor A spent about 30 minutes discussing various elements of the college search process, and asked if there were any questions at the end of group. There were none and the meeting ended. Counselor A decides that they need a new strategy before offering the next distance classroom guidance lesson.

DISCUSSION QUESTIONS

1. Reflect on Counselor A's planning process for the online classroom guidance lesson. What did Counselor A do well and what could have been improved?

2. Discuss Counselor A's decisions to involve parents, and then not involve parents, in the session. How might their presence or absence impact student learning?

3. Counselor A made the decision to record sessions. What procedures or protocols might have needed to occur before making this decision?

4. Consider Counselor A's teaching style. To what extent did Counselor A utilize quality standards for online instruction?

5. Assuming good intent, what did Counselor A do well?

CRITICAL QUESTIONS IN DECIDING TO PRACTICE

School counselors often have large caseloads and limited time. For some school counselors, the appeal of distance school counseling may include an ability to support ill or at-risk students, access parents, or simply interact more with students in relation to deadlines and required information. Students may be more likely to respond to a text than an email. They may benefit from a virtual session with a parent to walk them through a college application or Financial Aid form. While these elements sound appealing, there are risks to practicing virtual school counseling such as those discussed. Before deciding to embark on distance school counseling, here are some questions to consider.

1. What training do you have in DC? What training would you need before you started to offer distance school counseling services?

2. How would you define your student population? How accessible is technology for them? What modalities (e.g., videoconferencing, phone, email) would be appropriate?

3. What accommodations do you need to make for your students regarding their language abilities, cultural needs, and learning differences?

4. What policies are in place at your school regarding distance delivery of school counseling services? (Hint: If the answer is "none," start by gathering a team to create them.)

5. What services are you planning to provide via DC? Group counseling, individual counseling, career planning, classroom guidance, consultation, or others?

6. To what extent are you seeking to involve parents in distance services? What adjustments would you need to accommodate parents?

7. Does your school counseling office have a website? Is the information that is posted accessible to persons with disabilities and accommodate the cultural/linguistic needs of your community?

8. What boundaries will you establish to separate your work life from your home life if using DC? How will you communicate these boundaries to students and parents?

9. What practices are already in place at your school to provide for the confidentiality of your students and your students' records? What might need to change or improve if you use DC?

10. How prepared are you to address student and parent concerns about social media? How do you need to adapt your communication or outlook toward social media to connect with your students regarding its impact?

VOICES FROM THE FIELD

Distance Counseling With School Children

Cassandra Fleck, NCC, Certified School Counselor

I work as a counselor in a school setting with students in Pre-K through grade 12. It is a rural district with approximately 50% of students on a free or reduced lunch rate. As a school counselor, I provide tier 1 (social/emotional education), tier 2 (behavior plans and group counseling), and tier 3 (IEP counseling, crisis intervention, etc.) interventions. After the COVID-19 shut down we were suddenly forced to shift all counseling services to a distance format. On a Friday, I was sitting in my office with students and responding to classroom calls. By Monday, I was working from home.

This transition presented several challenges. The primary difficulty is navigating lack of access to the Internet in our community. There are many children for whom teleconferencing is not an option and we needed to do any counseling over the phone. This eliminates many body language cues and often children were uncomfortable talking on the phone. The disparities between our advantaged and disadvantaged families quickly became evident. Confidentiality also poses a challenge. We depend on adults to connect us with the younger children and support them with technology. Older students struggle to find a space away from siblings and other family members to talk. Many students don't have their own space and deal with everyday chaos in the home. Guardians try to limit this but it often creates more stress for them with poor results.

On the contrary, adolescents have gravitated toward email and text platforms. Some students have been more open and benefit from that lag time between responses to reflect and gain insight. Adolescents tend to be more comfortable with the technology and sometimes seem to prefer it over face-to-face interaction.

The unique aspect of utilizing DC for children is the reliance on parent support to connect with the child. In a school setting, all children have access to the school counselor. When using a distance format, we need to go through the parent to set the child up to speak with us. This results in increased involvement of parents but can also present challenges if a guardian is resistant or hard to reach. Some parents are trying to satisfy basic needs such as food and do not understand the role that counseling support can play.

For anyone considering using DC with children it is a necessity to be flexible and creative. Each family has access to different technologies so one session may be via teleconferencing, some via email, or others over the phone. The wide range of school counselor duties requires us to become comfortable recording ourselves to deliver tier 1 lessons. It requires creativity in how we connect with students. School counselors must ensure equal access for all children and this may mean the counselor needs to adapt for each family. Ways that we accomplished this were by sending encouraging notes, accommodating various schedules, delivering kindness rocks, and doing some virtual "lunches" that gave children time to relax and continue to build rapport without the expectation of working toward their goals.

STUDENT AFFAIRS COUNSELING

Student affairs professionals support college students in their personal development through a variety of roles and functions, including college counseling centers, academic advising, career counseling, student activities, residence life, veteran's affairs, and others. NASPA, formerly the National Association of Student Personnel Administrators, designates 36 Knowledge Communities (KC) that outline the unique specializations of student affairs professionals, including professionals serving Graduate Students, Adult Learners, African Americans, Alcohol and Other Drug, Disability, Fraternity Sorority, Gender and Sexuality, Indigenous Persons, International, Latnix/a/o, and many others (NASPA, n.d.). The American College Personnel Administration (ACPA), another professional development organization serving student affairs professionals, defines 18 Active Commissions, similar to NASPA KCs, including Housing and Residential Life, Recreation, Social Justice Education, Spirituality and Faith, Student Conduct, Two-Year Colleges, and many more (ACPA, 2018). A cursory review of NASPA's KCs and ACPA's Active Commissions demonstrate the breadth and depth of work in student affairs. The diversity of college students directly impacts the use of DC/TMH applications. As has been discussed, elements such as culture, age, geography, and socioeconomic status will impact an individual's access to technology, which in turn impacts their appropriateness for DC/TMH interventions.

Mental Health

The college process can have a significant impact on college students' mental health. The American College Health Association's National College Health Assessment (2019) found that approximately 40% of college students experienced moderate to serious psychological distress, and nearly 50% screened positive for loneliness. Additionally, the survey indicated that 9% of college students actively engage in self-injury or self-harm, 23% screen positive for suicidal behavior, and 2.4% of students attempted suicide within the past 12 months. College students indicated that their highest stressors were procrastination, academics, and finances, followed by intimate relationships, family, health of someone close to them, and career. For some college students, being away from home for the first time can add to feelings of stress and loneliness, particularly for residential students living far from home. Some college counseling centers may elect to provide DC/TMH services while students are on break or to students taking online classes. These centers would want to monitor any state telemental health laws for students living out of state, including laws where the student is located. As a registered student at the university, the student is likely eligible to receive counseling services. However, variations in state TMH laws should be reviewed to avoid potential conflicts.

Ethics

The professional counseling association that addresses college students is the American College Counseling Association (ACCA). While other professional counseling organizations develop ethical standards, ACCA supports the use of the Council for the Advancement of Standards (CAS) in Higher Education. CAS publishes standards for nearly 50 higher education specialties including Counseling Services (CAS, 2020). The CAS standards for Counseling Services Section 11 focuses on the use of technology in relation to college counseling settings. Specifically, Section 11.1, Systems Management, calls on college counseling services to provide current technology to support student development, and to incorporate technology in to their programs and services. The standards specify that staff be trained in technology, data be backed up regularly, and the college have a plan to keep technology current. Section 11.2, User Engagement, indicates that college counseling services use technology to enhance their services, meet client needs, and provide remote access. Section 11.3, Compliance and Information Security, requires that college counseling services follow laws and guidelines to protect client information, including financial transactions. Finally, Section 11.4, Communication, specifies that websites are current and accessible, communication formats are secure, technology and social media are used ethically, and that counseling services "evaluate multiple modes of communication, including but not limited to, phone, text, and web chat" (CAS, 2019, p. 24). These standards reflect content addressed earlier, such as ensuring counselors are trained to utilized TMH counseling, using secure and encrypted equipment, and ensuring that technology is accessible to all populations served.

College settings serve students in multiple capacities. College counseling centers are responsible for protecting students' health records, and must comply with the Health Insurance Portability and Accountability Act (HIPAA) guidelines, while also protecting electronic health information if using technology or electronic medical records (EMR). Other college services, however, such as Registrar and Academic Advising, are responsible for protecting students' academic records, and as such, must be sure to comply with the Family Educational Rights and Privacy Act (FERPA). Student affairs professionals must consider their obligation to protect student information and ensure that DC/TMH services comply with required federal and state guidelines. In a college setting, it is important to recognize that most students are legal adults, which may impact parents' access to both academic and medical records. Each university will have policies pertaining to waivers and parent access to medical and/or academic records; DC/TMH interventions will be required to follow these designated procedures.

Effectiveness

College populations have responded well to DC/TMH interventions in prior research. One reason for favorable DC/TMH outcomes may be college students' perceived barriers to accessing college counseling centers. Barriers to accessing college counseling centers may include stigma associated with receiving mental health care, lack of social support among peers, the students' inability to communicate their mental health needs effectively, as well as not seeing a need or not being ready to receive counseling support (Berman et al., 2019). Other barriers to accessing college counseling centers include travel time and cost, specifically for adults not living on campus, and concerns about seeing their counselor on campus outside of session (Simpson et al., 2015). Benefits of online college interventions include being cost-effective, increasing access to treatment, and providing services while students are on a wait list (Benton et al., 2016). College students engaging in TMH interventions reported feeling at ease in TMH sessions and feeling more control than in face-to-face (F2F) sessions, after getting over their initial adjustment to TMH services. College students also report that they were able to build a therapeutic alliance with their TMH counselor and that the TMH interventions were effective, even when working with counselors-in-training (Benton et al., 2016; Simpson et al., 2015). In a study which included online psychoeducation, homework, short-term counselor interactions via brief video sessions, and text reminders from the counselor, college students with anxiety actually experienced greater reduction in anxiety symptoms than those attending traditional F2F counseling (Benton et al., 2016). These outcomes may be due to the appeal and comfort of technology for college populations.

Mobile Applications

The appeal of technology also includes mobile applications, which is a topic that has not been fully addressed in this book. Mental health mobile applications, also known as "apps," are downloaded to a mobile device and may provide support for an individual's mental health and well-being. A variety of apps exist for mindfulness strategies, cognitive behavioral interventions, addictions, and other supports. Mobile apps are not addressed as a TMH modality in this book based on the limited interaction users have with a personal counselor. However, it should be noted that mobile apps, or e-interventions, are regularly utilized with college students for a variety of issues such as psychoeducation on alcohol and drug use, sexual assault, and other topics. As indicated in the Benton et al. (2016) study, mobile apps are being created, such as the treatment-assisted online (TAO) intervention for anxiety, that combine online psychoeducation with homework assignments, self-monitoring, and check-ins from an individual counselor. Other interventions include biofeedback devices and entering mental health data (e.g., cravings, negative thinking, or anxiety) on mobile devices in real time, as opposed to self-report at later weekly sessions. This real-time data can be reviewed by a counselor during individual sessions, including TMH sessions. These interventions differ from large scale e-interventions used at colleges and universities to reduce risky behavior, such as binge drinking. While these large scale e-interventions tend to be effective in reducing binge drinking in the short term, the impact of these interventions is reduced beyond 6 to 12 months after completing the intervention (Prosser et al., 2018). Recommended interventions for longer term support include wearable technology that monitors blood alcohol content (BAC), interactive gamification apps, and online platforms for peer support (Prosser et al., 2018).

CASE STUDY: STUDENT AFFAIRS

Counselor A is an academic advisor on a college campus, which serves primarily residential students. The academic advising center has a detailed, secure, self-service portal where students can log in and complete many academic functions, such as adding a class, dropping a class, withdrawing from a class, or requesting a grade exception. The academic advising center does not offer distance advising sessions as the portal allows students to access many functions 24 hours a day. Students are still required to meet with their advisor at least once a semester for academic advising, academic holds, major selection, and academic probationary issues. Counselor A works on a 12-month contract in the academic advising center.

Client B is a student completing sophomore year as a Chemistry major with the hopes of following the pre-Med curriculum. Client B recently returned home, out of state, and learned that they failed two classes, including organic chemistry, which is a requirement for the Chemistry major. After 2 years of academic difficulties, Client B is coming to terms with the fact that medical school is not likely. Client B emailed Counselor A asking for help in changing their fall schedule and possibly changing their major. Counselor A responded to the email explaining that a videoconferencing session would be best, such that they could look at Client B's transcript together, as well as academic plans for other majors. Client B responded to the email and agreed to the videoconference session, but also stated that they didn't want their parent to find out. Counselor A responded to the email with a secure link to the videoconference. They also explained in the email that some students find it easier to talk to their parents about their academic struggles, as opposed to trying to hide their academic struggles and parents finding out later. Client B wrote back, "not my parents—see you on the video call."

The morning of the videoconference Client B appeared on the screen with Parent C sitting next to them on camera. Client B did not look at the camera, but looked down at the ground. Counselor A greeted Client B, and asked if someone was going to be joining them for the call. Client B did not respond. Parent C stated,

> I am Client B's parent. I'm going to talk to you about what classes Client B needs to take to get into medical school. Client B told me that you told them to speak to me—so thank you for that. But Client B is going to be on the pre-Med track, and we are going to use this call to figure out how we can do that.

Client B continued to look away from the camera. Counselor A attempted to speak to Client B directly, and asked "Client B, do you want Parent C to be with us on the call today? I need your permission in order for us to discuss your academics with them." Parent C interrupted by saying, "I don't know what you are talking about. I'm the parent and of course I can be on the call. I remember some nonsense about this at freshman orientation but I had Client B sign the waiver so I can talk to you about grades." Counselor A is able to check Client B's records and notices that there is no current valid FERPA waiver on file. While Client B did sign the FERPA waiver before their freshman year, giving Parent C permission to discuss grades, they rescinded the waiver at the end of their freshman year after grades were posted.

DISCUSSION QUESTIONS

1.   What are your thoughts on Counselor A recommending a video session? What are the pros and cons to a video session in this scenario?

2.   How well did Counselor A prepare for the video session? If you were Counselor A, what other steps might you have taken before scheduling the video session?

3.   Spend some time thinking about Client B. What do you think this client may be going through, both when Client B reached out via email, and now on the video session? How would you be able to help via DC?

4. Spend some time thinking about Parent C. What do you think they may be going through, both after talking to Client B, and now on the video session? How would you be able to help via DC?

5. Assuming good intent, what did Counselor A do well?

CRITICAL QUESTIONS IN DECIDING TO PRACTICE

Student affairs and college counselors work in a wide variety of settings. The decision to utilize DC or TMH counseling in a college setting may be impacted by the professional role of the counselor. For example, services such as mental health counseling, academic advising, and career counseling may be more easily adapted to a TMH/DC modality, than residence life, student activities, or campus recreation specialists. Before considering the transition to DC/TMH interventions, it is critical to consider not only one's role with college students, but also the demographic of the students being served. Below are some additional questions to reflect on regarding distance services with college students.

1. What is your role in providing services to college students? How can that role effectively utilize DC/TMH interventions?

2. What is the population of students that you serve? Have you assessed their access, ability, and interest in using DC/TMH interventions?

3. What is your training in DC/TMH? How well prepared are you to offer DC/TMH services to students?

4. Consider the types of stressors that college students face – specifically the stressors that your students face. How can DC/TMH interventions address those concerns?

5. If you are a part of a college counseling office, how well does your office abide by the CAS standards outlined for technology?

6. What university polices or state/federal codes do you need to examine before offering DC/TMH services?

7. How might you need to adapt permission statements and informed consent documents if you were offering DC/TMH services?

8. How might you need to create or adapt policies for students living out of state?

9. What steps do you need to take to protect student information? Consider your office's obligation to adhere to HIPAA and/or FERPA guidelines.

10. How do students, faculty, and staff respond to help-seeking behaviors of students? What can you do – using DC/TMH – to reduce barriers for college students seeking help?

VOICES FROM THE FIELD: COLLEGE STUDENT COUNSELING

Telemental Health With College Students

Jennifer Yeager Lloyd, MA, NCC, LPC

Woodbridge Counseling, LLC, is a solo practitioner private practice located in rural northwestern Pennsylvania (Meadville, PA). I serve numerous college-aged students here, and it is in that capacity that I feel TMH has been most valuable for my practice.

The benefit of doing TMH for a college-aged population is that, once you have rapport established, these students do not have to feel like they will "lose ground" when they return home for the summer. I can offer continuity across settings as they choose. These students have also verbalized to me that they hesitate to use "on campus" services, as they don't like to run into their support staff while on campus or doubt the integrity of the confidential campus counseling process.

There are some occasional difficulties or limitations with the nature of rural WiFi/Internet. Some students must work with their technology departments to obtain special permissions, as the HIPAA protected platform I use, Virtualtherapyconnect.com (VTC), requires a considerable amount of bandwidth and signal strength. A signal can be weak and trouble with video or audio can ensue. Sometimes sessions can be interrupted by returning roommates or people walking through "The Quad" if a student is sitting outdoors. Many students have come up with creative alternatives such as sitting in their cars, driving to local stores that have better/free WiFi, or locating a secure spot on campus and using earphones to protect their audio.

I have faced one other considerable "snag" that anyone providing virtual therapy to college students should be aware of: Students may indicate they are engaging in self harm or feeling suicidal or homicidal. What do you do?

If you are considering doing virtual therapy with a college client base, be sure you have an Informed Consent that adequately explains how you will address self-harm, suicidal ideation, and homicidal ideation (and, of course, the possible technology limitations in general). You do not want to be caught in a moment where a student discloses something of a reportable nature without having informed them (and educated yourself) about what will occur.

TMH for college students has been fantastic for Woodbridge because the use of technology is "normal" for that age group. Most are accustomed to an online platform and have no issues switching between use of phone or laptop (and VTC provides apps for both!). They appreciate the convenience of not having to leave campus or being able to follow up with me throughout the summer.

I strongly suggest any counselor considering support of college students using TMH. Be sure to adequately explain limitations to your client base, as well as educate yourself about how to handle technology or safety issues that will arise.

CONCLUSION

DC and TMH have been effectively utilized with children, adolescents, and college-aged students. School counselors and student affairs counselors need to examine their role in providing services to students, and the capacity in which DC/TMH can enhance those services. In working with minors, counselors will want to focus on obtaining parental consent, in addition to minor assent, as well as the manner in which parents may be needed to facilitate DC interactions. Similarly, college settings will need to manage parental desire for involvement with students' rights. Both school and student affairs counselors must have appropriate training in DC/TMH service delivery and ethical concepts, including both HIPAA and FERPA, depending on context. Finally, school and student affairs counselors must know the population they serve, including their access to technology and their ability to use it. The ethical guides posted by the ASCA and CAS in College Counseling provide guidance to practitioners considering DC/TMH interventions.

REFERENCES

American College Health Association. (2019). *National College Health Assessment III Fall 2019 Reference Group Executive Summary.* https://www.acha.org/documents/ncha/NCHA-III_Fall_2019_Reference_Group_Executive_Summary.pdf

American College Personnel Administration. (2018). *Active commissions.* https://www.myacpa.org/commissions

American School Counselors Association. (2016). *ASCA ethical standards for counselors.* https://www.schoolcounselor.org/asca/media/asca/Ethics/EthicalStandards2016.pdf

American School Counselors Association. (2020). *School counseling during COVID-19: Online lessons and resources.* https://www.schoolcounselor.org/school-counselors/professional-development/learn-more/coronavirus-resources

Benton, S. A., Heesacker, M., Snowden, S. J., & Lee, G. (2016). Therapist-Assisted Online, (TAO) intervention for anxiety in college students: TAO outperformed treatment as usual. *Professional Psychology Research and Practice, 47*, 363–371. https://doi.org/10.1037/pro0000097

Berman, A., Bevan, J. L., & Sparks, L. (2019). Readiness to visit university counseling centers: Social support, stigma, and communication efficacy. *Journal of Student Affairs Research and Practice, 57*(3), 282–295. https://doi.org/10.1080/19496591.2019.1648272

Carlson, L. A., Portman, T. A. A., & Barlett, J. R. (2006). Professional school counselors' approaches to technology. *Professional School Counseling, 9*, 252–256. https://doi.org/10.5330/prsc.9.3.9162536405845454

Comer, J. S., Furr, J. M., Miguel, E. M., Cooper-Vince, C. E., Carpenter, A. L., Elkins, R. M., Kerns, C. E., Cornacchio, D., Chou, T., Coxe, S., DeSerisy, M., Sanchez, A. L., & Chase, R. (2017). Remotely delivering real-time parent training in the home: An initial randomized trial of Internet-delivered Parent-Child Interaction Therapy (I-PCIT). *Journal of Consulting and Clinical Psychology, 85*, 909–917. https://doi.org/10.1037/ccp0000230

Council for the Advancement of Standards in Higher Education. (2019). *Counseling services*. CAS Standards and Guidelines. https://www.cas.edu

Council for the Advancement of Standards in Higher Education. (2020). *Standards*. https://www.cas.edu/standards

Council on the Accreditation of Counseling and Related Education Programs. (2020). *Find a program*. https://www.cacrep.org/directory

Gallo, L. L., Rausch, M., & Wood, S. (2016–2017). School counselors' experiences working with digital natives: A qualitative study. *Professional School Counseling, 20*, 14–24. https://doi.org/10.5330/1096-2409-20.1.14

Groetzinger, K. (2020, April 22). *Navajo families without Internet struggle to home-school during COVID-19 pandemic*. NPR. https://www.npr.org/2020/04/22/839948923/navajo-families-without-internet-struggle-to-homeschool-during-covid-19-pandemic

International Society for Technology in Education. (2020). *ISTE Standards*. https://www.iste.org/standards

Joosten, T., Cusatis, R., & Harness, L. (2019). A cross-institutional study of instructional characteristics and student outcomes: Are quality indicators of online courses able to predict student success? *Online Learning Journal, 23*(4). https://doi.org/10.24059/olj.v23i4.1432

Kamenetz, A. (2019, October 31). *It's a smartphone life: More than half of U.S. children now have one*. NPR. https://www.npr.org/2019/10/31/774838891/its-a-smartphone-life-more-than-half-of-u-s-children-now-have-one

McCarty, C. A., Vander Stoep, A., Violette, H., & Myers, K. (2015). Interventions developed for psychiatric and behavioral treatment in the children's ADHD telemental health treatment study. *Journal of Child and Family Studies, 24*, 1735–1743. https://doi.org/10.1007/s10826-014-9977-5

NASPA. (n.d.). *Knowledge communities.* https://naspa.org/communities/knowledge-communities

Pennant, M. E., Loucas, C. E., Whittington, C., Creswell, C., Fonagy, P., Fuggle, P., Kelvin, R., Naqvi, S., Stockton, S., & Kendall, T. (2015). Computerized therapies for anxiety and depression in children and young people: A systematic review and meta-analysis. *Behaviour Research and Therapy, 67,* 1–18. https://doi.org/10.1016/j.brat.2015.01.009

Pew Research Center. (2019, June 12). *Internet/Broadband Fact Sheet.* https://www.pewresearch.org/internet/fact-sheet/internet-broadband

Prosser, T., Gee, K. A., & Jones, F. (2018). A meta-analysis of effectiveness of E-interventions to reduce alcohol consumption in college and university students. *Journal of American College Health, 66,* 292–301. https://doi.org/10.1080/07448481.2018.1440579

Pullen, S. J., White, J. O., Salgado, C. A., Sengupta, S., Takala, C. R., Tai, S., Swintak, C., & Shatkin, J. P. (2013). Video-teleconferencing with medical students to improve exposure to child and adolescent psychiatry. *Academic Psychiatry, 37,* 268–270. https://doi.org/10.1176/appi.ap.12040073

Osborn, D. S., Peterson, G. W., & Hale, R. R. (2015). Virtual school counseling. *Professional School Counseling, 18,* 179–190. https://doi.org/10.5330/2156-759X-18.1.179

Prensky, M. (2001). *Digital natives, Digital immigrants.* https://www.marcprensky.com/writing/Prensky%20-%20Digital%20Natives,%20Digital%20Immigrants%20-%20Part1.pdf

Schaeffer, K. (2019, August 23). *Most US teens who use cellphones to it pass time, connect with others, learn new things.* Pew Research Center. Fact Tank: News in the Numbers. https://www.pewresearch.org/fact-tank/2019/08/23/most-u-s-teens-who-use-cellphones-do-it-to-pass-time-connect-with-others-learn-new-things

Siegler, K. (2020, April 24). *Even in crisis times, there is a push to wire rural America.* NPR. https://www.npr.org/2020/04/24/843411430/even-in-crisis-times-there-is-a-push-to-wire-rural-america

Simpson, S., Guerrini, L., & Rochford, S. (2015). Telepsychology in a university psychology clinic setting: A pilot project. *Australian Psychologist, 50,* 285–291. https://doi.org/10.1111/ap.12131

Steele, T. M., Jacokes, D. E., & Stone, C. B. (2015). An examination of the role of online technology in school counseling. *Professional School Counseling, 18,* 125–135. https://doi.org/10.5330/prsc.18.1.428818712j5k8677

Stephan, S., Lever, N., Bernstein, L., Edwards, S., & Pruitt, D. (2016). Telemental health in schools. *Journal of Child and Adolescent Psychopharmacology, 26,* 266–272. https://doi.org/10.1089/cap.2015.0019

Taylor, D. B. (2020, May 5). How the corona pandemic unfolded: A timeline. *The New York Times.* https://www.nytimes.com/article/coronavirus-timeline.html

Troung, D. (2020, March 18). *As classes move online, what happens to students without Internet or computers?* NPR. https://www.npr.org/local/305/2020/03/18/817691597/as-classes-move-online-what-happens-to-students-without-internet-or-computers

Wilczenski, F. L., & Coomey, S. M. (2006). Cyber-communication: Finding its place in school counseling practice, education, and professional development. *Professional School Counseling, 9,* 237–331. https://doi.org/10.5330/prsc.9.4.78t6014366615205

10

Specialized Areas of Practice: Clinical Populations and Telemental Health

INTRODUCTION

The telemental health (TMH) movement emerged from telehealth and telepsychiatry movements beginning in the 1960s and expanding through the 1990s (American Psychiatric Association [APA], n.d.). Through these early interactions, TMH was often used in the assessment and treatment of mental illness. Similarly, Alcoholics Anonymous (AA) first utilized distance groups in the 1960s, with a variety of distance group modalities expanding in to the 1990s (AA, 2020). While AA represents a peer support group and not a counseling group, the utility of distance counseling (DC) via support groups has been widely utilized by the recovery community. Clinicians have successfully treated mental illness and addictions with DC/TMH in a multitude of research studies. Professional counseling associations, such as the American Mental Health Counselor Association (AMHCA) and NAADAC (formerly the National Association for Alcohol and Drug Addiction Counselors), provide guidance to mental health and addictions counselors on the use of DC/ TMH interventions with the clients they serve.

CLINICAL MENTAL HEALTH COUNSELING

Licensed mental health counselors utilize a variety of professional titles including Licensed Clinical Mental Health Counselor (LCMHC), Licensed Mental Health Counselor (LMHC), Licensed Professional Counselor (LPC) and others (AMHCA, 2020). Mental health counselors are committed to the emotional and mental health of individuals, and "assess, diagnose, and treat mental disorders defined in the *Diagnostic and Statistical Manual of Mental Disorders*" (AMHCA, 2020, p. 3). This treatment may be delivered in a variety of settings including inpatient hospitals, partial hospitalization programs, outpatient clinics, and private practices (Gerig, 2018). The *Diagnostic and Statistical Manual of Mental Disorders, Fifth Edition (DSM-5)* provides a framework of diagnostic criteria to assist mental health practitioners in making a diagnosis and determining the need for treatment. As specified in the *DSM-5*, the presence of a diagnosis does not necessitate a need for treatment (APA, 2013), however for some individuals, the impact of their mental health disorder may warrant clinical treatment. Research has demonstrated that TMH interventions have been effective with a variety of mental health diagnoses, including those addressed in the following.

Evidence-Based Telemental Health Interventions in Clinical Mental Health Counseling

The *DSM-5* is categorized into over 20 broad diagnostic categories including neurodevelopmental, schizophrenia spectrum, bipolar, depressive, anxiety, obsessive-compulsive, trauma, somatic, feeding/eating, elimination, sleep-wake, sexual, gender dysphoria, impulse control, substance-related, neurocognitive, personality, paraphilic, and other related disorders. Within these broad diagnostic categories, there are a multitude of individual mental health diagnoses and specifiers for these diagnoses (APA, 2013). While TMH research may not have been conducted on every diagnosis and condition identified in the *DSM-5*, there are a multitude of common diagnoses that have been repeatedly evaluated and effectively treated with TMH interventions.

Posttraumatic Stress Disorder

Researchers have adapted traditional face-to-face (F2F) interventions used to treat posttraumatic stress disorder (PTSD) to TMH interventions. Using clinical interventions such as prolonged exposure (PE) therapy (Yuen et al., 2015), behavioral-activation and therapeutic exposure (BA-TE; Acierno et al., 2016), and psychoeducation on emotion management and interpersonal regulation skills (Weiss et al., 2018), studies have found that TMH performed no worse than F2F interventions in reducing PTSD symptoms. TMH had a greater impact on reducing symptoms of PTSD among veterans (Acierno et al., 2016), which may be related to veterans being less likely to seek counseling in a F2F setting. A great deal of research has been conducted on the use of TMH interventions with military members diagnosed with PTSD. This is likely due to the fact that PTSD is a common mental illness among military members who have experienced trauma, or that military organizations, such as the Veterans Administration (VA), have access to a large number of patients diagnosed with PTSD. It should be noted that much of the data surrounding the effectiveness of PTSD and TMH have been published by VA researchers and may not be generalizable beyond military populations.

Depression

Much of the research focused on depression and TMH utilizes Internet-based cognitive behavioral therapy (iCBT) interventions. These interventions include a variety of formats including self-paced, self-help instructional models; psychoeducation and homework; and supportive feedback from a therapist via distance modalities (El Alaoui et al., 2016; Hedman et al., 2011; Rosso et al., 2016). While these iCBT studies have indicated overall positive success rates in treating depression, the attrition and dropout rates for these programs vary. A meta-analysis of iCBT research on clients with depressive symptoms revealed that clients complete iCBT interventions less frequently than those in traditional treatment (van Ballegooijen et al., 2014). Research has demonstrated that adherence to iCBT treatment significantly impacts symptom reduction (El Alaoui et al., 2016). These iCBT interventions appear to be effective across genders and across age groups (Hobbs et al., 2018). Patients utilizing iCBT improved in other areas of functioning, such as sleep disorders (El Alaoui et al., 2016; Hedman et al., 2011) and suicidal ideation, while also maintaining improved depressive symptoms at 6-month followup (Hedman et al., 2014a). In addition, iCBT interventions have been utilized with special populations experiencing depressive symptoms, including pregnant women (Forsell et al., 2017) and persons with late-life depression (Hobbs et al., 2018). While iCBT interventions have been effective in reducing depressive symptoms, researchers recognize the need for increased interactions with counselors (Mathiasen et al., 2016). There are concerns that much of the research on iCBT has been published by those who developed the iCBT interventions (Arnberg et al., 2014).

It is important to address suicidality when discussing TMH depression interventions. Suicide risk is increased with a variety of mental health conditions including depression and mood disorders (APA, 2013). Many of the iCBT studies include reduced therapist contact and use of self-help, self-paced interventions, which do not provide for emergency crisis intervention. However it should be noted that the majority of these research studies excluded participants who were experiencing active suicidal ideation or were at risk for suicide. For counselors using TMH intervention, such as iCBT or other distance modalities, it is prudent to include protocols and procedures for emergency contact when the client is experiencing suicidal thinking (Rosso et al., 2016). As has been previously addressed, the need to develop detailed informed consent procedures, emergency protocols, and safety plans are a critical component of any TMH intervention, regardless of diagnosis or presenting symptomology.

Anxiety

The use of iCBT also permeates the literature pertaining to TMH and anxiety. A multitude of studies have examined the use of iCBT interventions on generalized anxiety disorder (GAD; Lorian et al., 2012), social anxiety (El Alaoui et al., 2015; Hedman et al., 2011; Hedman et al., 2014b), and health-related anxiety (Gross et al., 2017; Soucy & Hadjistavropoulos, 2017). The use of iCBT did reduce anxiety symptoms in some studies (Hedman et al., 2014b; Morris et al., 2016) but not all (Gross et al., 2017; Lorian et al., 2012). Interestingly, computer or technology anxiety may reduce the effectiveness of iCBT interventions for individuals experiencing anxiety disorders (Soucy & Hadjistavropoulos, 2017). While iCBT has been found to be effective in reducing anxiety symptoms for individuals on wait lists, there is less evidence to support its efficacy when compared to F2F treatment (Arnberg et al., 2014). Beyond iCBT, anxiety has been treated effectively with videoconferencing and the use of Family Cognitive Behavioral Therapy (Carpenter et al., 2018). There is also evidence that the use of text-based services may eliminate barriers to treatment for individuals with symptoms of anxiety (Nitzburg & Farber, 2019).

A multitude of other mental health disorders have been addressed using TMH research, including obsessive compulsive disorder, eating disorders, and suicidality. These studies examine the impact of interventions, such as videoconferencing, telephone, iCBT alone, iCBT supported by a therapist, and the use of mobile applications or "apps," to reduce symptoms of mental illness. Mobile apps are utilized to address a variety of mental health conditions including anxiety reduction, mood disorders, anger management, eating disorders, and others (Parker et al., 2018). Mobile apps are often used as a complement to F2F or TMH counseling. TMH counseling has been praised as an opportunity to expand the work of private practitioners (Neuer Coburn, 2013). Like all TMH interventions, using TMH in mental health counseling requires adherence to ethical codes and practice standards.

Ethical Issues in Clinical Mental Health Counseling and Telemental Health

The AMHCA provides clear and comprehensive guidelines for the mental health counselor engaging in TMH. The AMHCA Code of Ethics (2015), Section 6. Telehealth, Distance Counseling, and the Use of Social Media, outlines several parameters specific to DC/TMH interventions. The AMHCA begins by stating that mental health counselors recognize the value technology brings to mental health care, and to "engage in technology assisted, or distance counseling" (p. 10). This standard implies that technology will be a standard component of all mental health counseling practice, at least to some extent. The AMHCA codes specify that the counselor using TMH be licensed in the same state as the client, excluding emergency treatment, and that even in emergencies the counselor attempts to gain permission from the state (6a). The AMHCA requires counselors engaging in TMH to have training and experience in TMH (6b), as well as written policies, addressing email, text, online scheduling, and chatrooms (6c). The AMHCA discourages the use of chatrooms due to the inability to assist in a crisis situation.

Safety continues to be a primary ethical concern. The AMHCA requires counselors to follow safety guidelines, protect clients from interruptions, and utilize local resources in an emergency (6d). Counselors are responsible for determining if a client is appropriate for TMH services (6e), and also to conduct themselves in a professional manner during online counseling sessions "as if the client were in the counselor's office" (6d; p. 11). In accordance with safety procedures, counselors must inform all clients about the safety and security of records (6e). This includes their responsibility to protect client records, and to prohibit session recordings on the part of the counselor or client. Recordings can only be authorized with consent and must be destroyed in a timely manner. Safety also involves the use of social media. The AMHCA clearly states that counselors "do not engage in virtual relationships with clients" (6h; p. 11). Specifically, these policies require that counselors have separate social media profiles for personal and professional accounts, not solicit professional reviews by clients, and only conduct Internet searches on clients to determine the client's health or safety.

The AMHCA also requires counselors to be aware of cultural differences, including disabilities, in the same manner as they would if they were conducting F2F sessions (6i). These specific guidelines in Section 6, are offered alongside the AMHCA's overall guidelines that address the mental health counselor's commitments to clients, other professionals, students, supervisees, employees, the profession, and the public. These commitments to practice ethically and effectively must be balanced with the laws that govern TMH practice, and the regulations of managed care.

Telemental Health and Managed Care

The practice of licensed mental health counseling is overseen by the licensing boards of each state issuing a license to a mental health practitioner. Professional counseling licensure now includes all 50 states in the United States, as well as the District of Columbia, Puerto Rico, and Guam, and is managed by 53 separate entities (American Counseling Association [ACA], 2020). Licensure laws for mental health providers vary from state to state (Epstein Becker Green Law, 2019). This book has earlier addressed the importance of technological security and encryption, as well as adherence to the Health Insurance Portability and Accountability Act (HIPAA) guidelines and safeguarding electronic protected health information (e-PHI) of clients. However, many mental health counselors utilize insurance reimbursement and electronic billing, which adds an additional layer of caution and scrutiny for TMH practice.

Malpractice Insurance

Most mental health counselors carry malpractice insurance, either through their employer or their own policy. For the counselor who is providing TMH services, it is important to confirm that one's malpractice insurance also covers TMH sessions (Luxton et al., 2016). The counselor should be sure that their insurance covers them for TMH sessions in both the state that they are located in, as well as the state that their client is located in. While the AMHCA (2015) codes specify that counselors only provide services when they are licensed in the state of the clients, state laws may differ (Epstein Becker Green Law, 2019). Thus, counselors may face a situation in which their ethical codes and state laws conflict. For these reasons, it is critical that counselors' malpractice insurance covers TMH interventions in any state where the client or counselor is located. The counselor should also confirm that their insurance covers them for supplemental tasks, such as supervision or consultation. Some malpractice insurance companies consider supervision as a separate function that requires additional coverage. If those tasks are being conducted remotely, it is prudent to verify that malpractice covers those services whether delivered remotely or in-person.

Insurance Reimbursement and Billing

Many mental health counselors are reimbursed for services via a client's insurance company. A mental health provider can join one or several insurance panels as a means of serving clients who hold that insurance. The client pays a copay to the provider, and the provider will submit documentation to the insurance company for reimbursement. When delivering TMH services, the provider is responsible for confirming if that insurance provider will reimburse for TMH services. Services are identified via Current Procedural Terminology (CPT) codes (American Academy of Professional Coders, 2020), and specific CPT codes are utilized when services are provided via telemental health. Previously, insurance companies may have elected to reimburse for one modality, such as videoconferencing, and not another, such as telephone. Medicaid and Medicare had strict guidelines for TMH reimbursement (Luxton et al., 2016). In the weeks following the COVID-19 stay-at-home order, insurance reimbursement for TMH services, and all telehealth services, seemed to change overnight. Amid the COVID-19 closures, many insurance companies committed to TMH reimbursement and lifted restrictions for telehealth and TMH services. As of this writing, these policies are currently in place, but there is no indication of how long these policies will remain. The counselor is advised to ensure that TMH services are covered by any insurance company that they plan to seek reimbursement from for TMH services.

Integrative Healthcare

According to the Substance Abuse and Mental Health Services Administration (SAMHSA), people with mental health disorders and addictions struggle with a variety of medical conditions and are more susceptible to early death than those without mental health disorders and addictions (SAMSHA, n.d.). Through the integrative healthcare initiative, individuals receive care for all conditions in one health setting, such as their primary care provider. Individuals have the ability to address both their physical and emotional wellness, as opposed to navigating multiple obstacles to treatment. TMH can play an active role in supporting integrative health care initiatives. Integrative healthcare is about connecting clients to services and eliminating barriers to treatment. TMH has been effective in helping at-risk groups gain access to treatment, such as rural populations, veterans, people with disabilities, and those unlikely to seek treatment. Counselors have an opportunity to provide TMH services to persons with addictions and/or mental health disorders by collaborating with integrative health professionals.

CASE STUDY: CLINICAL MENTAL HEALTH COUNSELING

Counselor A is a licensed mental health counselor who has decided to expand their practice by participating in a major turnkey counseling platform. Through this platform, the company reviews Counselor A's license and malpractice insurance, and connects Counselor A only to clients that the counselor is licensed to serve. Being located in New York, Counselor A assumes that they are only connected to clients in New York, although they do not confirm client locations once assigned. Counselor A engages primarily in message-style counseling, in which they communicate with clients only via a messaging feature within the platform. The platform is secure and encrypted according to the company's website. Through this platform, Counselor A creates an informed consent document, but did not create an emergency plan because the company collects emergency contacts for every client they serve. When a new client is presented to Counselor A, the counselor is provided with the client's presenting problem statement and the counselor can then elect to accept the client or not. Counselor A's client issues range from mild to moderate depression and anxiety, primarily focused on presenting concerns such as loneliness and relationships. One client, Client B, had articulated that they were an international student, but they were enrolled in a college in New York. Client B explained that the distance from home was contributing to their loneliness. Counselor A was unsure about providing treatment to international students, however, but because the student was enrolled in a New York college, the counselor assumed Client B was covered under their New York license.

Counselor A had been successfully working with clients for approximately one month when they received a request for a new client, Client C. Client C's presenting statement indicated that they were a resident of an Asian country and were located in that country at the time of their contact. In their presenting statement, Client C indicated active suicidal ideation, stating that "every day I want to die" and "I know exactly how I would kill myself but I'm too scared to do it." Counselor A was alarmed by the request, both based on the content of the presenting problem and the client's international location. Counselor A's immediate reaction was to click on the "identify emergency contact" option, however when doing so, they were prompted with a warning message to make sure the client was in danger and that they were not violating the client's confidentiality by notifying emergency contacts. Because Client C was not yet Counselor A's client, the message caused Counselor A pause and they did not notify the emergency contact.

Instead, Counselor A immediately contacted the company via their messaging system to explain the situation. Counselor A explained that they were uncomfortable accepting this client, as well as the concern that the client appeared to be in danger. Counselor A also asked how this client was assigned to them being that they are located out of the country. The company responded immediately, stating that Counselor A did not need to accept the client and that they would proceed to assign the case to another counselor and manage the emergency situation. The company explained that there is a setting in Counselor A's profile that allows them to accept international clients, and that if they don't wish to serve international clients, they should deselect that option.

DISCUSSION QUESTIONS

1. What training does Counselor A have in TMH? How might this impact their practice?

2. How do you feel about how Counselor A set up the TMH practice? What other actions might have been helpful, either from Counselor A or the company?

3. Consider Counselor A's interactions with Client B. What are your thoughts on how they handled that case? How might it have been improved, if at all?

4. Consider Counselor A's interactions with Client C. What are your thoughts on how they handled that case? How might it have been improved, if at all?

5. Assuming good intent, what did Counselor A do well?

CRITICAL QUESTIONS IN DECIDING TO PRACTICE

Mental health counselors are likely to experience a demand for TMH services, particularly following the COVID-19 pandemic. Counselors may have quickly adapted to TMH services without a thorough reflection on the necessary elements for a successful and ethical practice. The following questions provide an opportunity for reflection for the mental health counselor considering implementing TMH services.

1. What training, experience, and supervision do you have in TMH counseling? If none, how can you obtain this training and supervision prior to practice?

2. What is the population that you are planning to serve via TMH? Are there any additional precautions needed when using TMH with this population?

3. Consider the entirety of the AMHCA Ethical Codes. How well does your practice adhere to these codes? What will you need to change or improve to engage in ethical practice?

4. Where will you and your clients be located? Are you licensed where your clients are located? If not, are you willing to seek licensure in those states?

5. What are the licensing laws for providing TMH both in your state and the state in which your clients are located? Are (or will you be) in compliance with these laws?

6. Does your malpractice insurance cover TMH practice? If not, are you willing to pay additional premiums for TMH coverage?

7. Will you be engaging in any additional clinical services, such as supervision or consultation via TMH? If so, does your malpractice insurance cover those activities?

8. What insurance panels are you on? Do you know if they reimburse for TMH services?

9. When was the last time you reviewed your insurance panel's TMH reimbursement policies? Have they changed recently due to COVID-19?

10. What integrated care initiatives exist in your area? Is there an opportunity for you to support these initiatives with your TMH practice?

VOICES FROM THE FIELD: CLINICAL MENTAL HEALTH COUNSELING

TMH Treatment in Mental Health Counseling

Tyce Nadrich, PhD, LMHC, ACS, NCC

I am a part-time clinician in a private practice who shares space with two colleagues. Prior to TMH, my practice day was Sundays and I would see anywhere between 4 to 8 clients in a day. I work predominantly with adolescents and adults of color. Also, I typically have counseling interns in my office, so I do supervision with them and occasionally join in on their sessions.

Shifting my practice to include TMH offered both advantages and limitations. The largest and most salient advantage is accessibility. I am much more accessible to my clients via TMH; clients are no longer required to travel and I can offer more flexibility in scheduling since I do not have to worry about office space. I do not want to understate the importance of accessibility. Being more accessible is significant to clients, and it allows me to serve those I may not have been able to with my limited office hours and location.

Although there are multiple challenges to TMH, the most salient to my practice include clinical assessment, technological difficulties, and reimbursement. All clinicians must do thorough assessments with their clients to both understand their needs and ensure their safety. When engaging via TMH, I found clinical assessment more difficult due to changes in administration procedures and crisis response. I have had to alter how I complete my standardized assessments to not distribute documents illegally. Consequently, I must either read the assessment to my client or display it via screen sharing and record their verbal answers. The process is comparatively untimely and far less seamless compared to an in-person

assessment. Additionally, if a client's results are indicative of harmful ide-
ations, I may have to spend extra time with the client to ensure their safety.
Logistically, when practicing in person, the process was fairly simple: I
would walk out to my waiting room, let my next client know I'm running
late, and return to the session. However, via TMH, I must call, email, or
text my next client (which they may not see or answer), and now edit my
sessions within my TMH platform to ensure all the video portals are accessible and correct. This is not unmanageable, but a different kind of work
compared to in-person counseling.

Technology and reimbursement also present unique challenges when
engaging in TMH counseling. I am fairly tech savvy, so my computer
can effectively handle video conferencing and I have sufficient Internet
speeds. However, some clients may lack the knowledge of technology to
ensure their devices or Internet speeds are capable, or may lack the means
to acquire the necessary technology. This can result in a poor connection
to the therapy session, resulting in other challenges. Further, not all insurance companies include TMH in their contracts. As such, you may need to
apply for privileges to provide TMH services, which can be untimely and/
or laborious, assuming you are granted the privilege at all.

One unique aspect of my TMH practice is managing distractions with/
for clients. Most of my clients are lower to middle class. As such, they frequently do not have private spaces within their homes to attend counseling
sessions uninterrupted. My office afforded comparatively unparalleled privacy. Sometimes my clients will have their family, pets, or even the doorbell
interrupt their sessions. Further, when working with adolescents, they are
easily distracted by their environment. They are trying to attend counseling
in the same place where they live their lives; there are a myriad of distractions, from their devices, books, and hobbies, to their family and friends.
This is certainly not a deal breaker, and I do not believe this challenge
supersedes the paramount importance of increased accessibility. Nevertheless, it is a challenge the counselor and client must overcome together.

The best advice I can offer counselors preparing to offer TMH services
through their private practice is preparation and rules. Do your homework
on the TMH platforms you can use to provide services, ensuring their pric-
ing is fair and they offer Health Insurance Portability and Accountability
Act compliant access. Communicate with your insurance panels to confirm
you will receive compensation for providing TMH services. Also, confirm
the procedures and codes required for billing, as they may be different
from in-person sessions. Prepare for the transition as much as possible,
but also be prepared to learn as you transition. Establish rules with your
clients to help them transition, too. Have open conversations with them
about TMH and how it will affect your work together. Allow them to ask
any questions about TMH and create a document that you can share with
them so they can process everything on their own time. Lastly, speak with

them about what makes TMH counseling effective and model effective session dynamics, as you would for in-person counseling.

ADDICTION COUNSELING

According to SAMHSA's 2018 National Survey on Drug Use and Health, approximately 19.3 million adults in the United States have a substance use disorder. This number includes the approximately 9.2 million adults with both a substance use disorder and a mental illness (SAMHSA, 2019), also known as having a co-occurring disorder. Addiction counseling is a specialization recognized by the Council on the Accreditation of Counseling and Related Education Program (CACREP); however, based on the large percentage of individuals with co-occurring disorders, many mental health counselors also obtain credentials and experience in substance use counseling. The *DSM-5* classifies substance use disorders (SUD) into ten substance categories including alcohol, caffeine, cannabis, hallucinogens, inhalants, opioids, sedatives, stimulates, tobacco, and other substances. Within these categories, a client may meet criteria for various disorders and levels of severity (APA, 2013). Beyond substances, a variety of behaviors may classify as addictive behaviors, sometimes referred to as process addictions (Smith, 2015). Gambling disorder is the first process addiction to be included in the *DSM* under nonsubstance disorders (APA, 2013), however a variety of other behaviors may be considered addictive including sexual activity, disordered eating, work addiction, exercise addiction, compulsive shopping/buying/spending, and Internet use (Smith, 2015). Specialized trainings and certifications have been developed to assist counselors in treating certain process addictions, such as gambling and sexual addiction.

Individuals experiencing SUD and process addiction will require treatment, much like those with other mental health disorders. Like those with mental health disorders, individuals with SUD and process addictions may also experience stigma or shame associated with seeking treatment. DC and TMH have been known to assist individuals to gain access to treatment, while also minimizing the stigma associated with treatment (Avent Harris et al., 2020; Neely-Fairbanks et al., 2018). Unlike receiving face-to-face (F2F) treatment, individuals receiving DC/TMH treatment do not need to visit a substance use treatment facility, and may not need to take time off from their work or responsibilities in order to attend treatment. In addition, TMH has been found to be effective in connecting people in rural communities to treatment (Imig, 2014; Lambert et al., 2016; Mehrotra et al., 2017; Weiss et al., 2018), indicating that TMH can provide support to rural areas impacted by opioid, methamphetamine, and other drug crises.

Evidence-Based Telemental Health Interventions in Addictions

Addictions research that focuses on the use of TMH is also heavily weighted with iCBT interventions. Specifically, iCBT interventions have been utilized to manage addictions to smoking (Smit et al., 2016), cocaine (Schuab et al., 2011), and gambling (Carlbring et al., 2012). Like iCBT research on depression and anxiety, iCBT research with addictions demonstrates moderate effectiveness, yet low completion rates. Similarly, mobile apps have emerged to assist in the treatment of other addictions, such as alcohol (Barrio et al., 2017). Like iCBT, the use of mobile apps may involve therapist intervention via messaging, email, text, or video sessions, or may be a standalone service without counselor intervention. A meta-analysis focusing on self-help interventions for alcohol use, drug use, and smoking found that, while self-help interventions can be beneficial, clients achieve and maintain greater outcomes with the intervention of a professional counselor (Newman et al., 2011). Thus, the use of iCBT and mobile apps in TMH addictions treatment does not eliminate the role of professional counselors.

Counselors have successfully utilized videoconferencing with motivational interviewing strategies to address high risk alcohol use and sexual behavior (Celio et al., 2017). Videoconferencing has been utilized for medication assisted treatment (MAT) in rural communities, with positive outcomes for those who persisted in the program (Weintraub et al., 2018). Videoconferencing has successfully been utilized to manage co-occurring disorders in veterans with PTSD (Jaconis et al., 2017). Substance use treatment facilities appear to have both an interest and commitment to using technology. In a study of over 350 substance abuse facilities, facilities most frequently indicated that they were using computerized screening and assessment (44%), telephone-based recovery support (29%,) telephone-based therapy (28%), and video-based therapy (20%). However, these facilities' interests in technology included computerized screening/assessment (69%), text app reminders (68%), web portals for patients (58%), mobile apps (55%), and video-based therapy (54%; Molfenter et al., 2018, p. 3). These numbers indicate that there is both a desire and potential to increase TMH interventions in SUD treatment facilities.

SUD treatment is underutilized, often due to limited access or stigma affiliated with seeking help. It would be logical to assume that TMH interventions could assist in access, reduce cost, and increase immediacy of substance use treatment, as well as reduce stigma. Technology provides additional supports to clients outside of treatment sessions (Molfenter et al., 2018). However, barriers exist to accessing addiction treatment via TMH. In a study of 1.9 million health insurance records, the number of people diagnosed with SUD increased nearly five times between 2010 and 2017 (2010 = 0.62/1K, 2017 = 3.05/1K). During this same time period, the number of telehealth visits also increased nearly 18 times its starting rate (2010 = 0.91/1K, 2017 = 16.59/1K). However, despite these increases, TMH-SUD visits only accounted for 1.4% of all telehealth visits (Huskamp et al., 2018). These findings illustrate that, at the time of this writing, TMH utilization in SUD remains low. Addictions counselors are encouraged to explore opportunities to use DC/TMH interventions that are effective, appropriate, and ethical.

Ethical Issues in Addictions and Telemental Health

The professional counseling organization for addiction counselors is the International Association of Addictions and Offenders Counseling (IAAOC), which is a division of the ACA. As has been discussed in this book, the ACA publishes detailed ethical codes outlining practices for both F2F and DC/TMH interactions. Many addiction counselors elect to join NAADAC: The Association for Addiction Professionals, formerly known as the National Association of Alcohol and Drug Abuse Counselors. Like the ACA and the AMHCA, NAADAC publishes a Code of Ethics (2016) that specifies practice for addiction counseling, including Principle VI: E-Therapy, E-Supervision, and Social Media. This section of the NAADAC code outlines 20 areas of practice for addictions counselors providing DC/TMH interventions.

NAADAC includes both e-therapy and e-supervision in its code and begins with a reminder to use HIPAA-compliant technology (Section VI-1). Counselors must have training and competence in DC/TMH interventions prior to practice (VI-2). Similar to the ethical codes of other counseling specializations, NAADAC outlines content to be included in the Electronic/Technology informed consent, and specifies that the language must be clear and understandable, as well as reviewed verbally and in writing with clients (V-3 and VI-4). Counselors must verify client identity during DC/TMH sessions (VI-5) and adhere to all state and federal licensing laws pertaining to DC/TMH services (VI-6 and VI-7). NAADAC specifies that counselors must warn clients about the use of nonsecure technology, and also that therapy should not occur via text or email (VI-8). Counselors must assess a client's ability to benefit from DC/TMH interventions (VI-9), and also inform clients of other professionals who have access to their technology (VI-10).

Counselors are required to inform clients when they are working as part of a multidisciplinary team (VI-11), and also be aware of local resources near the client should the counselor need to make a referral for in-person services (VI-12). Counselors are required to maintain professional boundaries in distance relationships (VI-13), discussing these boundaries, as well as the potential to miss cues during DC/TMH services (VI-15). Counselors must assess the client's ability to use the technology, including their cognitive, developmental, and linguistic capabilities (V-14). Counselors must also understand the risks of electronic medical records (EMR) and make efforts to protect EMR (VI-16) in compliance with all state and federal laws (VI-17). Finally, in relation to social media, NAADAC specifics that counselors will not accept requests from clients to connect via social media, will keep separate social media accounts for personal and private use (VI-19), and will explain social media policies to clients (V-20).

No discussion of ethics and confidentiality in addiction treatment would be complete without addressing Title 42, Code of Federal Regulations, Part 2, sometimes referred to as "Title 42 CFR Part 2," or simply "Part 2." Part 2 is a federal law that was designed to protect the confidentiality of records of patients who received substance use treatment. Thus, any program that receives federal funds is required to comply with Part 2. Part 2 is designed to ensure that a client who is "receiving treatment for a substance use disorder in a part 2 program is not made more vulnerable by reason of the availability of their patient record than an individual with a substance use disorder who does not seek treatment" (Federal Register, 2017, p. 6053). A critical component of Part 2 is receiving written consent to transmit any client data, as well as not disclosing information without written consent of the client.

The use of EMRs and DC/TMH may increase the risk of security breaches and unintentional disclosure of information. These unintentional violations may occur when transmitting client information via email, or utilizing Internet-based platforms to send and receive information. In the weeks following the COVID-19 closures, SAMHSA issued a statement that, due to the shelter-in-place orders, providers may not be able to obtain written consent to release information. SAMHSA also specified that, in the case of a medical emergency, a provider may be able to disclose client information only to the extent that the client is in need of emergency medical treatment (SAMHSA, 2020). As has been addressed in this book, DC/TMH requires the use of a safety plan, including emergency contacts and local emergency information. For the addictions counselor providing DC/TMH interventions, it would be reasonable to include a consent document on what client information can be released in these emergency situations, as well as how the counselor can/should define their relationship to the client, in case of emergency. Due to Part 2 regulations, a counselor whose facility is receiving federal funds may not disclose a client's participation in substance use treatment without written consent.

Finally, client safety continues to be a primary concern in any TMH practice, including addictions counseling. The disease of SUD poses significant risk to client safety, including medical risks associated with intoxication, overdose, and withdrawal. NAADAC codes (2016) regularly address the need for collaboration and working as a part of a multidisciplinary team. Access to medical providers may be a critical component of addiction treatment, including the need for medication assisted treatment (MAT), managing withdrawal, and prescribing psychiatric medication for clients with co-occurring disorders. Addiction counselors need to maintain these collaborative relationships in distance settings. Counselors may need to establish preferred medical protocols for psychiatric evaluation, medication evaluation, referral to a higher level of care, or obtaining required toxicology testing. Distance modalities may limit the counselor's ability to notice small cues such as tics or odor that could signify a greater medical concern, such as adverse reactions to medication or relapse. Counselors need to make plans to address these potential medical risks, and include plans for addressing relapse and medical emergencies both in informed consent documents and emergency planning.

CASE STUDY: ADDICTIONS

Counselor A is an addiction counselor at an outpatient substance use treatment facility. At the facility, Counselor A conducts group and individual counseling, intakes, and documentation. Counselor A is responsible for calling clients who miss their treatment appointments, and encouraging them to attend treatment. About half of the clients at the facility are mandated to treatment due to substance-related criminal activity or issues regarding family/parenting. Counselor A has been working with Client B for approximately 3 months as the primary counselor. Through this role, Counselor A has weekly individual sessions with Client B, develops and updates the treatment plan, and communicates with Client B's probation officer on the treatment. Counselor A also collects toxicology samples (drug tests) to monitor Client B's abstinence from drugs and alcohol.

Client B has a diagnosis of alcohol use disorder, severe (F10.20), in early remission, as the client attended a 90-day residential program prior to outpatient treatment. During individual sessions, Client B has been working on attending 12-step meetings, obtaining a sponsor, and gaining employment. Client B regularly attends 12-step groups, weekly counseling, and has tested negative for drugs and alcohol. Client B recently got a job at a local hotel as a porter. The hotel is attached to a casino where there is excessive drinking among guests. Counselor A and Client B discussed the risk of this job in relation to relapse. Client B stated awareness of the triggers, had developed coping strategies, and plans to attend meetings.

Counselor A explained that Client B would need to continue the treatment due to the court mandate, and offered weekly individual videoconferencing sessions. The agency has a secure, encrypted counseling platform and has trained all staff in telemental health. Client B reported that they did not want to do a video session because "I don't want you to see my place." Counselor A offered phone sessions through the software platform, but explained that Client B would need to come in and provide weekly toxicology samples when the facility was open. Client B agreed to this arrangement, and signed a detailed informed consent with an emergency plan.

Client B initially participated in weekly phone sessions, usually from their car, before or after a work shift, and also provided regular toxicology samples. During one of these sessions, Client B shared that they had met a romantic partner at work. Counselor A knew from prior sessions that relationships were contributing factor to Client B's relapse history. When confronted, Client B stated that they knew the triggers and had coping strategies; Client B reported that they had not been able to attend 12-step meetings due to the work schedule. When Client B did not attend a scheduled session, Counselor A called to follow-up. Client B stated that they could not talk because they had their romantic partner in the car and had "forgot" about the session. Counselor A called Client B after their shift to discuss their attendance. Client B became aggravated and angry, telling Counselor A to stop "hassling me" and "leave me be." Counselor A discussed how, in their previous sessions, Client B shared that anger and yelling could be an indication of relapse. Counselor A mentioned that Client B had not provided a toxicology sample in 3 weeks, at which point, Client B hung up the phone.

DISCUSSION QUESTIONS

1. Discuss the agency and Counselor A's preparation for TMH sessions. Which aspects of preparation were strengths, and which, if any, could have been improved?

2. Counselor A had the opportunity to meet with Client B in person before transitioning to TMH. How was that either an asset or a liability in this case?

3. Client B is mandated to treatment. How might the client's mandate impact the use of TMH services, if at all?

4. Consider Client B's reactions. What might Client B be experiencing, and how can Counselor A or the agency assist?

5. Assuming good intent, what did Counselor A do well?

CRITICAL QUESTIONS IN DECIDING TO PRACTICE

Addiction counselors have an opportunity to expand access to SUD treatment, and possibly minimize some of the stigma of receiving treatment by engaging in TMH practice. Yet preparing for TMH practice requires preparation and planning. Following are some areas to consider when adapting your present addiction counseling practice to a TMH modality.

1. What training do you have in TMH? Per NAADAC standards, do you have additional certifications and/or courses, supervision, and experience in TMH?

2. What type of modalities will you use to deliver services? Consider NAADACs statement on not allowing therapy via email or text in your decision.

3. How will you determine if clients have the capabilities to utilize the technology you select? How will you assess intellectual, emotional, and linguistic competence?

4. What is the population of clients you serve and what is their access to technology? If you serve mandated clients, what adaptations might you need?

5. Consider the entirety of the NAADAC code of ethics, not simply Section VI. How well does your practice adhere to the ethical standards outlined?

6. Will you utilize any EMR systems? How will you confirm the security of the client records you keep?

7. Consider Title 42 CFR Part 2 if you are receiving federal funding. How might you need to share client information? Consider additional consents that need to be developed.

8. Research demonstrates that clients who persist in TMH treatment have better outcomes in recovery. What are some ways you can continue to keep clients engaged in treatment?

9. Counselor involvement also contributes to successful client outcomes. How can you maximize involvement in TMH while maintaining boundaries?

10. Many people who are in need of SUD treatment do not seek treatment due to stigma associated with addiction. How can you create a TMH practice that reduces stigma and promotes the value of SUD treatment?

VOICES FROM THE FIELD: ADDICTIONS COUNSELING

Treating Addictions via Technology

Jessica L. Auslander, MA, LCMHC, LCAS, ICGC-I, NCC/NCSC, BC-TMH

I provide TMH services to clients in three states over the phone or via web-based secure portal. I am independently licensed in clinical mental health, addiction, and certified in the treatment of gambling disorder. Many of my cases begin as "telesupport." These are employee assistance program (EAP) clients who continue services utilizing their insurance; most were not aware that TMH existed beyond the EAP program.

One of the significant benefits of practicing TMH with this population is being able to remove barriers to services. Clients often comment that they prefer TMH because it offers them more control over their care and privacy. They do not have to leave their homes or explain why they need to leave work for an appointment. They do not need to get themselves "ready" to be in public or handle the stress of public interaction. They do not have to spend time commuting to an office or miss appointments due to lack of transportation. A significant challenge to working with those affected by addiction through telehealth is that it limits the range of services one can provide. The intake process must be done very carefully to ensure that distance services are truly the most appropriate fit for the client. If a client has a medical emergency or needs a higher level of care, the counselor must be prepared to facilitate the transition; therefore, it is vital to research emergency and referral resources in the client's area at the beginning of treatment. One unique aspect of doing TMH with this population is working with clients who are seeking treatment for gambling, gaming, Internet use, or any other disorder or behaviors that rely on technology for access. In these cases, the device that was often used in the illness now becomes part of the treatment. Addressing the client's relationship with technology can provide additional insight that might inform creative interventions.

To professionals considering engaging in TMH with this population, I would strongly suggest pursuing certification. I was initially certified in 2005 as a Distance Credentialed Counselor (offered by the NBCC) because I was a school counselor at an online charter school. As my career has evolved I have maintained this certification (now BC-TMH). It's more than knowing how to integrate technology into your practice; there are constantly evolving legal and ethical considerations that must be considered, addressed, and documented in your professional disclosure statement. Carefully consider your reasons for providing TMH services as well as your own level of comfort. For some clients, it may be appropriate to only offer it on a limited basis to prevent a missed appointment, while for others it may be their only option due to geographical distance or other barrier. As with any other technique or treatment modality, we must regularly engage in continuing education, supervision, or consultation, and stay within the boundaries of our competence.

CONCLUSION

The professions of Clinical Mental Health Counseling and Addictions Counseling continue to grow. According to the Bureau of Labor Statistics (BLS), mental health and substance abuse counseling jobs are expected to grow 22% by 2028 (BLS, 2020). As these fields grow within the counseling profession and the use of TMH expands, clinical mental health counselors and addiction counselors will be integrating technology into their daily practice. Research supports the use of TMH to treat both mental health and SUDs. While much of the research is focused on the use of iCBT and mobile apps, there is concern about clients' treatment adherence with these self-paced modules. In addition, evidence demonstrates that the role of the counselor enhances clinical outcomes, specifically, the use of videoconferencing. Like all TMH practice, clinical mental health and addictions counselors are guided by the ethics of the profession, including the AHMHCA and NAADAC codes of ethics. For clinical mental health counselors, particular cautions of TMH practice involve managed care, billing, and insurance; however, there are opportunities to expand TMH in to integrative care settings. Addiction counselors must also concern themselves with 42 CFR Part 2 regulations that protect client confidentiality, as well as the need for collaboration with the medical community to support client safety.

REFERENCES

Acierno, R., Gros, D. F., Ruggiero, K. J., Hernandez-Tejada, B. M. A., Knapp, R.G., Lejuez, C. W., Muzzy, W., Frueh, C. B., Egede, L. E., & Tuerk, P. W. (2016). Behavioral activation and therapeutic exposure for post- traumatic stress disorder: A noninferiority trial of treatment delivered in-person versus home based telemental health. *Depression and Anxiety, 33*, 415–423. https://doi .org/10.1002/da.22476

Alcoholics Anonymous. (2020). *Over 80 years of growth*. Timeline view. https:// www.aa.org/pages/en_US/aa-timeline/to/1

American Academy of Professional Coders. (2020). *What is CPT®?* https://www .aapc.com/resources/medical-coding/cpt.aspx

American Counseling Association. (2020). *Licensure and certification – State professional counselor licensure boards.* https://www.counseling.org/knowledge

-center/licensure-requirements/state-professional-counselor-licensure-boards

American Mental Health Counselors Association. (2015). *AMHCA code of ethics.* http://www.amhca.org/learn/ethics

American Mental Health Counselors Association. (2020). *Essentials of the clinical mental health counseling profession.* http://www.amhca.org/learn/ethics

American Psychiatric Association. (n.d.). *Telepsychiatry tool kit: History of telepsychiatry.* https://www.psychiatry.org/psychiatrists/practice/telepsychiatry/toolkit/history-of-telepsychiatry

American Psychiatric Association. (2013). *Diagnostic and statistical manual of mental disorders* (5th ed.). Author.

Arnberg, F. K., Linton, S. J., Hultcrantz, M., Heintz, E., & Jonsson, U. (2014) Internet-delivered psychological treatments for mood and anxiety disorders: A systematic review of their efficacy, safety, and cost-effectiveness. *PLoS ONE, 9*(5), e98118. https://doi.org/10.1371/journal.pone.0098118

Avent Harris, J. R., Crumb, L., Crowe, A., & Garland McKinney, J. (2020). African American's perceptions of mental illness and preferences for treatment. *Journal of Counselor Practice, 11*(1), 1–22. https://doi.org/10.22229/afa1112020

Barrio, P., Ortega, L., Lopez, H., & Gual, A. (2017). Self-management and shared decision-making in alcohol dependence via mobile app: A pilot study. *International Journal of Behavioral Medicine, 24,* 722–727. https://doi.org/10.1007/s12529-017-9643-6

Carlbring, P., Degerman, N., Jonsson, J., & Andersson, G. (2012). Internet-based treatment of pathological gambling with a three-year follow-up. *Cognitive Behaviour Therapy, 41*(4), 321–335. https://doi.org/10.1080/16506073.2012.689323

Carpenter, A. L., Pincus, D. B., Furr, J. M., & Comer, J. S. (2018). Working from home: An initial pilot examination of videoconferencing-based cognitive behavioral therapy for anxious youth delivered to the home setting. *Behaivor Therapy, 49,* 917–930. https://doi.org/10.1016/j.beth.2018.01.007

Celio, M. A., Mastroleo, N. R., DiGuiseppi, G., Barnett, N. P., Colby, S. M., Kahler, C. W., Operario, D., Suffoletto, B., & Monti, P. M. (2017). Using video conferencing to deliver brief motivational intervention for alcohol and sex risk to emergency department patients: A proof-of-concept pilot study. *Addiction Research & Theory, 25,* 318–325. https://doi.org/10.1080/16066359.2016.1276902

El Alaoui, S., Ljótsson, B., Hedman, E., Kaldo, V., Andersson, E., Ruck, C., Andersson, G., & Lindefors, N. (2015). Predictors of symptomatic change and adherence in internet-based cognitive behaviour therapy for social anxiety disorder in routine psychiatric care. *PLoS ONE. 10*(4), e0124258. https://doi.org/10.1371/journal.pone.0124258

El Alaoui, S., Ljótsson, B., Hedman, E., Svanborg, C., Kaldo, V., & Lindefors, N. (2016). Predicting outcome in Internet-Based Cognitive Behaviour Therapy for major depression: A large cohort study of adult patients in routine psychiatric care. *PLoS ONE, 11*(9), 1–16. https://doi.org/10.1371/journal.pone.0161191

Epstein Becker Green Law. (2019). *Telemental Health Laws [mobile application software].* https://play.google.com/store

Federal Register. (2017, January 8). *Department of Health and Human Services*. Office of the Secretary. 42 CFR Part 2. Confidentiality of substance use disorder patient records. https://www.govinfo.gov/content/pkg/FR-2017-01-18/pdf/2017-00719.pdf

Forsell, E., Bendix, M., Hollandare, F., Szymanska von Schultz, B., Nasiell, J., Blomdahl-Wetterholm, M., Eriksson, C., Kvarned, S., van der Linden, J. L., Söderberg, E., Jokinen, J., Wide, K., & Kaldo, V. (2017). Internet delivered cognitive behavior therapy for antenatal depression: A randomized controlled trial. *Journal of Affective Behavior, 221*, 56–64. https://doi.org/10.1016/j.jad.2017.06.013

Gerig, M. S. (2018). *Foundations for clinical mental health counseling: An introduction to the profession* (3rd ed.). Pearson.

Gross, C. R., Reilly-Spong, M., Park, T., Zhao, R., Gurvich, O. V., & Ibrahim, H. N. (2017). Telephone adapted Mindfulness-based Stress Reduction (tMBSR) for patients awaiting kidney transplants. *Contemporary Clinical Trials, 57*, 36–43. https://doi.org/10.1016/j.cct.2017.03.014

Hedman, E., Andersson, E., Ljotsson, B., & Andersson, G. (2011). Cost-effectiveness of internet-based cognitive behavioral therapy vs. cognitive behavioral group therapy for social anxiety disorder: Results from a randomized controlled trial. *Behaviour Research and Therapy, 49*, 729–236. https://doi.org/10.1016/j.brat.2011.07.009

Hedman, E., Ljotsson, B., Kaldo, V. Hesser, H., El Alaoui, S. Kraepelien, M., Andersson, E., Rück, C., Svanborg, C., Andersson, G., & Lindefors, N. (2014a). Effectiveness of internet-based cognitive behavior therapy for depression in routine psychiatric care. *Journal of Affective Disorders, 155*, 49–59. https://doi.org/10.1016/j.jad.2013.10.023

Hedman, E., El Alaoui, S., Lindefors, N., Andersson, E., Ruck, C., Ghaderi, A., Kaldo, V., Lekander, M., Andersson, G., & Ljótsson, B. (2014b). Clinical effectiveness and cost-effectiveness of Internet- vs. group- based cognitive behavior therapy for social anxiety disorder: A 4-year follow-up of a randomized trial. *Behaviour Research and Therapy, 59*, 20–29. https://doi.org/10.1016/j.brat.2014.05.010

Imig, A. (2014). Small but mighty: Perspectives of rural mental health counselors. *The Professional Counselor, 4*, 404–412. https://doi.org/10.15241/aii.4.4.404

Hobbs, M. J., Joubert, A. E., Mahoney, A. E. J., & Andrews, G. (2018). Treating late-life depression: Comparing the effects of internet-delivered cognitive behavior therapy across the lifespan. *Journal of Affective Disorders, 226*, 58–65. https://doi.org/10.1016/j.jad.2017.09.026

Huskamp, H. A., Busch, A. B., Souza, J., Uscher-Pines, L., Rose, S., Wilcock, A., Landon, B. E., & Mehrotra, A. (2018). How is telemedicine being used in opioid and other substance use disorder treatment? *Health Affairs, 37*, 1940–1947. https://doi.org/10.1377/hlthaff.2018.05134

Jaconis, M., Santa Ana, E., Kileen, T. K., Badour, C. L., & Back, S. E. (2017). Case-series: Concurrent treatment of PTSD and alcohol use disorder via telehealth in female Iraq veteran. *The American Journal on Addiction, 26*, 112–114. https://doi.org/10.1111/ajad.12481

Lambert, D., Gale, J., Hartley, D., Croll, Z., & Hansen, A. (2016). Understanding the business case for telemental health in rural communities. *Journal of Behavioral Health Services & Research, 43*, 366–379. https://doi.org/10.1007/s11414-015-9490-7

Lorian, C. N., Titov, N., & Grisham, J. R. (2012). Changes in risk-taking over the course of internet-delivered cognitive behavioral therapy treatment for generalized anxiety disorder. *Journal of Anxiety Disorders, 26*, 140–149. https://doi.org/10.1016/j.janxdis.2011.10.003

Luxton, D. D., Nelson, E. L., & Maheu, M. M. (2016). *A practitioner's guide to telemental health: How to conduct legal, ethical, and evidence-based telepractice.* American Psychological Association.

Mathiasen, K., Andersen, T. E., Riper, H., Kleiboer, A. A., & Roessler, K. K. (2016). Blended CBT versus face-to-face CBT: A randomized non-inferiority study. *BMC Psychiatry, 16*, 432. https://doi.org/10.1186/s12888-016-1140-y

Mehrotra, A., Huskamp, H. A., Souza, J., Uscher-Pines, L., Rose, S., Landon, B. E., Jena, A. B., & Busch, A. B. (2017). Rapid growth in mental health telemedicine use among rural Medicare beneficiaries, wide variation across states. *Health Affairs, 36*, 909–917. https://doi.org/10.1377/hlthaff.2016.1461

Molfenter, T., Brown, R., O'Neill, A., Kopetsky, E., & Toy, A. (2018). Use of telemedicine in addiction treatment: Current practices and organizational implementation characteristics. *International Journal of Telemedicine and Applications*, Article ID 3932643, 7 pages. https://doi.org/10.1155/2018/3932643

Morris, J., Firkins, A., Millings, A., Mohr, C., Redford, P., & Rowe, A. (2016). Internet-delivered cognitive behavior therapy for anxiety and insomnia in a higher education context. *Anxiety, Stress, & Coping, 29*, 415–431. https://doi.org/10.1080/10615806.2015.1058924

NAADAC: The Association for Addiction Professionals. (2016). *Code of ethics.* https://www.naadac.org/code-of-ethics

Neely-Fairbanks, S. Y., Rojas-Guyler, L., Nabors, L., & Banjo, O. (2018). Mental illness knowledge, stigma, help-seeking behaviors, spirituality, and the African American church. *American Journal of Health Studies, 33*, 162–174. http://www.va-ajhs.com/33-4/index.aspx

Newman, M. G., Szkodny, L. E., Llera, S. J., & Przeworski, A. (2011). A review of technology-assisted self-help and minimal contact for drug and alcohol abuse and smoking addiction: Is human contact necessary for therapeutic efficacy? *Clinical Psychology Review, 31*, 178–186. https://doi.org/10.1016/j.cpr.2010.10.002

Neuer Coburn, A. A. (2013). Endless possibilities: Diversifying service options in private practice. *Journal of Mental Health Counseling, 35*, 198–210. https://doi.org/10.17744/mehc.35.3.8870230745378517

Nitzburg, G. C., & Farber, B. A. (2019). Patterns of utilization and a case illustration of an interactive text-based psychotherapy delivery system. *Journal of Clinical Psychology, 75*, 247–259. https://doi.org/10.1002/jclp.22718

Parker, L., Bero, L., Gillies, D., Raven, M., Mintzes, B., Jureidini, J., & Grundy, Q. (2018). Mental health messages in prominent mental health apps. *Annals of Family Medicine, 16*, 338–342. https://doi.org/10.1370/afm.2260

Rosso, I. M., Killgore, W. D. S., Olson, E. A., Webb, C. A., Fukanaga, R., Auerbach, R. P., Gogel, H., Buchholz, J. L., & Rauch, S. L. (2016). Internet-based cognitive behavioral therapy for major depressive disorder: A randomized controlled trial. *Depression & Anxiety, 34*, 236–245. https://doi.org/10.1002/da.22590

Schuab, M., Sullivan, R., & Stark, L. (2011). Snow Control – An RCT protocol for a web-based self-help therapy to reduce cocaine consumption in problematic cocaine users. *BMC Psychiatry, 11*(1), 153–160. https://doi.org/10.1186/1471-244X-11-153

Soucy, J. N., & Hadjistavropoulos, H. D. (2017). Treatment acceptability and preferences for managing severe health anxiety: Perceptions of internet-delivered cognitive behavior therapy among primary care patients. *Journal of Behavior Therapy and Experimental Psychology, 57*, 14–24. https://doi.org/10.1016/j.jbtep.2017.02.002

Smit, E. S., Candel, M. J. J. M., Hoving, C., & de Vries, H. (2016). Results of the PAS Study: A randomized controlled trial evaluating the effectiveness of a web-based multiple tailored smoking cessation program combined with tailored counseling by practice nurses. *Health Communication, 31*, 1165–1173. http://dx.doi.org/10.1080/10410236.2015.1049727

Smith, R. L. (2015). *Treatment strategies for substance and process addictions*. American Counseling Association.

Substance Abuse Mental Health Services Administration. (n.d.). *What is integrated care?* https://www.integration.samhsa.gov/about-us/what-is-integrated-care

Substance Abuse Mental Health Services Administration. (2019). Key substance use and mental health indicators in the United States: Results from the 2018 National Survey on Drug use and Health. *HHS Publication No. PEP19-5068.* https://www.samhsa.gov/data/sites/default/files/cbhsq-reports/NSDUH NationalFindingsReport2018/NSDUHNationalFindingsReport2018.pdf

Substance Abuse Mental Health Services Administration. (2020, March 19). *COVID-19 Public Health Emergency Response and 42 CFR Part 2 Guidance.* https://www .samhsa.gov/sites/default/files/covid-19-42-cfr-part-2-guidance-03192020.pdf

U.S. Bureau of Labor Statistics. (2020, April 10). *Occupational outlook handbook: Substance abuse, behavioral disorder, and mental health counselors.* https://www .bls.gov/OOH/community-and-social-service/substance-abuse-behavioral -disorder-and-mental-health-counselors.htm

van Ballegooijen, W., Cuijpers, P., van Straten, A., Karyotaki, E., Andersson, G., et al. (2014) Adherence to internet-based and face-to-face cognitive behavioural therapy for depression: A meta-analysis. *PLoS ONE, 9*(7), e100674. https://doi.org/10.1371/journal.pone.0100674

Weintraub, E., Greenblatt, A. D., Chang, J., Himelhoch, S., & Welsh, C. (2018). Expanding access to Buprenorphine treatment in rural areas with use of telemedicine. *The American Journal of Addiction Studies, 27*, 612–617. https://doi.org/10.1111/ajad.12805

Weiss, B. J., Azevedo, K., Webb, K., Gimeno, J., & Cloitre, M. (2018). Telemental health delivery of Skills Training in Affective and Interpersonal Regulation (STAIR) for rural women veterans who have experienced military sexual trauma. *Journal of Traumatic Stress, 31*, 620–625. https://doi.org/10.1002/jts.22305

Yuen, E. K., Gros, D. F., Price, M. Ziegler, P., Tuerk. P. W., Foa, E. B., & Acierno, R. (2015). Randomized controlled trial of home-based telemental health versus prolonged exposure for combat related PTSD in veterans: Preliminary results. *Journal of Clinical Psychology, 7*, 500–513. https://doi.org/10.1002/jclp.22168

11

Specialized Areas of Practice: Relationships and Life Transitions via Telemental Health

INTRODUCTION

Every person experiences life transitions. Transitions are life events that alter "our roles, relationships, routines, and assumptions" (Schlossberg, 2011, p. 139). These may include transitions into and out of work roles, relationship roles, family roles, and others, such as navigating life with a disability. These transitions may be planned and expected, or sudden and unexpected. They may be seamless or stressful, and many people require support during these transitional periods. In these circumstances, individuals may seek professional counseling from specialists such as Marriage, Couple, and Family counselors or Rehabilitation counselors. Like other counseling specializations, clients seeking support with transitions may benefit from the use of distance counseling (DC) and telemental health (TMH) counseling in order to access treatment. DC/TMH counseling allow individuals to access specialized counselors that have unique qualifications or clinical expertise, including linguistic abilities or experience with specific conditions. Similar to other counseling specializations, marriage, couple, and family counselors, as well as rehabilitation counselors, must adhere to professional ethical practice guidelines in order to competently serve their clients via DC/TMH modalities.

MARRIAGE, COUPLE, AND FAMILY COUNSELING

Marriage, couple, and family counseling is a Center for the Accreditation of Counseling and Related Education Programs (CACREP, 2016) specialization focusing on relationships, couples, and family systems. Marriage, couple, and family counseling is often confused with Marriage and Family Therapy (MFT). Marriage and Family Therapy is a profession that is distinct from professional counseling; MFT education programs are accredited by the American Association of Marriage and Family Therapy (AAMFT), not CACREP. The professional license for MFTs is the License in Marriage and Family Therapy (LMFT). MFT views work with couples and families as a profession in and of itself. Conversely, for marriage, couple, and family counselors, the professional license continues to be the Licensed Professional Counselor (LPC), or other titles, such as Licensed Mental Health Counselor (LMHC). Working with couples and families is viewed as a specialty within the counseling profession, similar to the specializations of school counseling, career counseling, rehabilitation counseling, and others. "Couple and family counselors advocate for the family as a whole system while considering the uniqueness of each family member" (IAMFC, 2017, p. 1). The professional counseling organization for marriage, couple, and family counselors is International Association of Marriage and Family Counselors (IAMFC).

Work with couples and families requires the coordination of multiple clients, and at times coordinating the schedules of working adults, along with the school and activity schedules of children and adolescents. It has been argued that the use of DC/TMH interventions can reduce the strain on clients to attend sessions, while also increasing the attendance rates of certain groups, such as men and adolescents, who are often hesitant to attend family and couples counseling (Doss et al., 2017). Professional counselors have successfully utilized DC/TMH interventions with marriage, couple, and family clients for a variety of clinical, personal and transition issues.

Evidence-Based Telemental Health Interventions in Couple and Family Counseling

Couple and family counseling succumbs to the same challenges as other counseling specializations. Clients in need of counseling services may struggle to obtain services due to geographic location, cost, stigma, or accessibility to services. To address these challenges, researchers have begun to utilize DC/TMH interventions as a way to bridge the gap between providers and needed services.

Military families face a variety of stressors including multiple relocations, extended absences of primary caregivers, as well as fear and anxiety for the military member's safety. Steven A. Cohen Military Family Center at NYU Langone Health in New York City piloted a TMH service in 2016 to expand their treatment to military member families and veterans (Price et al., 2018). Many clients began at the face-to-face (F2F) clinic for marriage and family therapy, but were recommended to TMH sessions for a variety of reasons. Some of these reasons included being unable to travel due to illness, work/family schedule, as well as subway anxiety. For one participant, TMH was the only type of therapy that they would accept. Depending on the presenting concern, counselors utilized a variety of therapeutic interventions via a secure video platform, including narrative therapy, exposure therapy, psychoeducation, and referral to a higher level of care. Participants described the at-home therapy as allowing them to have "freedom" and "control over their environment" (p. 274). In a related study, Families Over-Coming Under Stress (FOCUS), a military home visit program for families with preschool children, was successfully adapted to a DC/TMH model. Through this TMH intervention, counselors provided in-home virtual visits to parents alone, as well as joint parent–child sessions. These sessions provided guidance, psychoeducation on deployment and reintegration, development of a family narrative, and parenting skills to enhance the parent–child relationship (Mogil et al., 2015). The ability to visit a family home remotely was essential to treating Reservists and National Guard member families, many of whom live in the civilian community, miles away from military bases where services are traditionally offered.

Parent and child TMH interventions have been successful beyond the military community. Videoconferencing was used with family-based therapy (FBT) for adolescents with anorexia and their parents. Through an average of 20 sessions over a 6-month period, adolescent participants were able to increase their body mass index (BMI) to a healthy level, and maintain a healthy BMI at 6-month posttreatment follow-up (Anderson et al., 2017). Eating disorders are an example of a counseling specialization that requires clinical expertise, and TMH can provide access to families seeking qualified providers. Parent–child interaction therapy (PCIT) has been utilized as a parent training program for children with disruptive behavior disorders. PCIT was adapted to a home-based videoconferencing modality where parents used a headset to hear directives from the therapist, while interacting with their child. This format mimics traditional PCIT in which the therapist remotely monitors parent–child interactions, and provides feedback to parents via a bug-in-the-ear device. The study demonstrated that clients responded well to both PCIT and Internet PCIT (IPCIT; Comer et al., 2017). Much like Mogil et al.'s report (2015), this study provided parent–child training to parents of preschool children. Any parent of a preschool child can describe the struggle of getting their preschooler out of the house, let alone arriving at an appointment on time. The use of TMH with this population eliminates the stress on parents of transporting their preschool-aged child outside of the home, and increases the likelihood that the child will be comfortable using TMH in their own home. Additionally, early intervention can be critical to a child's development and behavior prior to entering a school setting.

Internet-based cognitive behavioral therapy (iCBT) has also been utilized in parent–child training programs; iCBT may include standalone self-help, self-paced training modules, or may involve counselor interventions. In a study of adolescents with chronic pain and their parents, use of an iCBT intervention was compared to a web-based psychoeducation program. Results indicated small, yet significant reductions in pain for the iCBT group, but no differences in the intensity of the pain (Palermo et al., 2016). iCBT has also been utilized with family caregivers of individuals with dementia (Blom et al., 2013). Couples and parents have benefited from the use of DC/TMH interventions. Kersting et al. (2011) assigned parents who had experienced the death of a child during pregnancy to either a wait list for grief counseling or an iCBT intervention that addressed posttraumatic stress, grief, and depression. Through this 5-week intervention, iCBT participant rates of grief and posttraumatic stress were significantly lowered. Similar to eating disorders or chronic pain, grief counseling is a clinical specialization that may not be readily available in one's area. Even if services are available, the wait time for services may be excessive. In these cases, the use of an iCBT or TMH intervention may allow the client to experience improvements while waiting to see a professional counselor. Other Internet recommendations for couples counseling include relationship advice websites, Internet assessments, Internet enrichment interventions for satisfied couples, and Internet interventions for at-risk couples (Cicila et al., 2014).

Ethical Issues in Couples/Family Counseling and Telemental Health

The IAMFC publishes a professional code of ethics for its members with the most recent update being published in 2017. The IAMFC clarifies that its professional code of ethics is designed to supplement the American Counseling Association (ACA) Code of Ethics (2014). Similar to the ACA Code of Ethics, the IAMFC codes provide detailed guidance pertaining to the counseling relationship, client welfare, confidentiality, privacy, competence, professional responsibility, supervision, research, and other areas of practice. Working with couples and families requires an awareness of family and relationship systems, whether practicing in F2F or DC/TMH settings. This specialization includes the ability to advocate for families, promote autonomy and decision-making, but not make decisions for the family. Like group counseling, couple and family counseling expects adherence to confidentiality. However, that confidentiality may not be respected by members outside of the session. Consents must be obtained from all adult clients, as well as from parents or guardians of minor children (IAMFC, 2017). In support of integrative care and DC/TMH interventions, the IAMFC advocates for interdisciplinary relationships with other helping professionals including psychiatry, psychology, social work, or other counseling specialties.

The IAMFC (2017) dedicates a specific section of the codes to technology, namely Section I: Technology Assisted Couples and Family Counseling. The IAMFC codes begin by clarifying that couple and family counselors *may* use technology when it is deemed to be appropriate. This explanation varies from earlier language in the American Mental Health Counselors Association (AMHCA) codes specifying that counselors *engage* in technology-assisted counseling, which may be interpreted as more of a directive than an option. Like all other ethical codes pertaining to DC/TMH, the IAMFC requires that couple and family counselors adhere to all federal and state laws pertaining to technology-assisted counseling. The IAMFC also requires counselors to comply with all judicial guidelines pertaining to technology-assisted counseling, and to not practice beyond their jurisdiction. This use of the term "jurisdiction" is unique and implies that counselors explore not only state and federal laws, but also local laws that may impact their practice. The IAMFC requires that couple and family counselors inform clients in writing as to the technological risks of distance counseling in relation to confidentiality and record keeping. Counselors are required to assess their clients' ability to use technology, as well as assess if using technology assisted counseling would benefit clients. Counselors are directed to only use technology that they are familiar with, as well as ensure that all technology meets safeguards for protected health information (PHI). While the IAMFC does not specify training in DC/TMH, the codes do require counselors to "adhere to the most current American Counseling Association guidelines regarding technology assisted counseling" (IAMFC, 2017, p. 9). This is an important clarification since the ACA outlines several guidelines for DC, including knowledge and competence in DC, guidelines for informed consent, confidentiality, verification, relationship, records, and social media. While these statutes are not explicitly outlined in the IAMFC codes, their reference to the ACA code and, specifically the ACA's focus on DC, presupposes these guidelines for couple and family counselors.

CASE STUDY: MARRIAGE, COUPLES, AND FAMILY

Counselor A is a Licensed Professional Counselor who graduated from a CACREP program with a master's degree in Marriage, Couple, and Family Counseling. Counselor A works for an organization that provides support to teenage mothers and their children up to age 5. The organization is affiliated with a community public health center that provides in-person parenting classes to expecting parents, telephone well-visits during the first 2 years after birth, and parenting training via videoconferencing for parents of children aged 0 to 5. Counselor A's agency also provides preschool for children aged 3 to 5, however children must be potty-trained in order to attend. Counselor A provides wellness checks and parenting training as a parent advocate. Counselor A has been assigned to work with Client B. Client B is a 19-year-old, single parent with a 3-year-old child. Client B and their child live with Client B's biological parent and stepparent in safe and secure housing. Client B is participating in parenting training and specifically requested help with potty-training and responding to temper tantrums. Client B did not participate in prior services with the agency. Client B has a 32-hour per week job at a retail store, and the biological grandparent provides child care while Client B is at work. Client B is hoping to get the child into the preschool once potty-trained.

Parent training consists of 10 weekly video sessions that are 1 hour in length. Clients need to sign in to a secure, encrypted video platform, and have access to a sufficient Internet bandwidth to communicate on the platform. Clients sign a detailed informed consent document outlining technology risks, limits of confidentiality, and a safety plan. During the first video session, Client B arrived on time with the child and appeared ready to work on the lesson. During the video session, Counselor A noticed that Client B regularly glanced at the bedroom door and at times appeared nervous. At one point, Client B startled at the same time that Counselor A heard a slamming noise. When asked about the noise, Client B stated that it must have just been the wind, but continued to look nervously at the bedroom door. During the second video session, Client B again arrived on time with the child, but spoke very softly and continually prompted the child to be quiet. At one point, Counselor A heard yelling in the background. Client B picked up the child and whispered for the child to be quiet. When Counselor A asked if everything was okay, Client B shook their head "no," put a finger to their lips to indicate silence, and put the computer on mute. Counselor A was able to hear continued shouting in the background. Client B eventually took the call off mute and asked if they could end for the day.

At the next session, Counselor A asked Client B what had happened the week prior. Client B apologized and explained that their stepparent gets very angry and that "it's best not to make any noise and try to disappear when that happens." Client B went on to explain that their stepparent often yells or makes comments about Client B and the baby, complaining that Client B is "using up all the heat and food in the house, and using my biological parent instead of paying child care." Counselor A then asked Client B if the home was safe for them and their child. Client B stated, "Yes. My stepparent would never do anything ... just yells a lot; it scares me and I feel guilty. That's why I need to get my child into preschool and give my stepparent one less thing to yell about."

DISCUSSION QUESTIONS

1. What training and experience, if any, does Counselor A have in DC/TMH? How might that influence this situation?

2. Consider the employer and Counselor A's preparation for DC/TMH sessions. What elements are strengths? What elements could be improved?

3. Consider the case of Client B. As Counselor A, what concerns might you have about the case? How does the presence of a child impact your concerns, if at all?

4. Counselor A has training with couples and parenting. How could they use this training with Client B, the child, and the grandparents, if at all?

5. Assuming good intent, what did Counselor A do well?

CRITICAL QUESTIONS IN DECIDING TO PRACTICE

Professional counselors can develop a specialization in work with families and couples. This can be achieved through specialized education and experience in working with families and couples. Marriage, couple, and family counselors can benefit from using DC/TMH interventions with their clients, but must also consider the ethical guidelines of their profession. As they consider expanding their practice, counselors may wish to reflect on the following questions in order to decide if a DC/TMH practice is appropriate and feasible.

1. As always, what training do you have in DC/TMH counseling before expanding your practice to distance modalities?

2. As always, what TMH modalities will you use to offer treatment? Do you have access to secure, HIPAA-compliant technology?

3. What specific training do you have in marriage, couple, and family counseling? How would you provide evidence as to your clinical specialization with couples and families?

4. Describe your client base. How appropriate are their clinical needs for DC/TMH? What concerns would you have about using DC/TMH with your population?

5. What are the access needs of your clients? Consider if DC/TMH is appropriate for your clients based on their developmental, cultural, and socioeconomic needs.

6. How would you mitigate some of the concerns you have in relation to questions 4 and 5? How might you prepare your practice to address these concerns?

7. What are the federal, state, and local laws in your area that may impact your DC/TMH service delivery?

8. Consider the ethical codes of both IAMFC and ACA, in their entirety. How well does your practice adhere to the codes, including specifications for DC/TMH practice?

9. How would you alter your consent forms for DC/TMH delivery of couple and family sessions? How will you gain minor assent, as well as parent/guardian consent?

10. Couples and family work presents challenges to confidentiality. How will you prepare for and navigate those challenges in a DC/TMH environment?

VOICES FROM THE FIELD: MARRIAGE, COUPLE, AND FAMILY COUNSELING

Telemental Health in Family Counseling

Leslie Caba, Second Year Clinical Mental Health Counseling Graduate Student

I began my first semester of internship in January of 2020 working with individuals of all age groups. Less than 2 months later, I was placed in the position of doing TMH due to COVID-19 with clients I had only seen about one to four times at most. Doing TMH was very difficult at first, primarily because I was still in the learning process of my internship. I was learning how to use the computer program used by this clinic and all the requirements I had to follow with each individual client. When quarantine began, I had to re-learn everything I had learned in the last 2 months, but with the changes of TMH.

Providing services through TMH was much more difficult when it came to my younger group of clients. My clients are 5 and 6 years old; the majority of my phone sessions are with the parent, primarily because the child does not stay on the phone the entire session or refuses to be on the phone at all. This is a difficult process because it involves teaching the parents how to do what I would be doing with the client if we were in-person. Many times, I teach parents different interventions or techniques to try with the client and the parent does not do it. This makes the treatment process difficult because the parent is the only way you can help this child and if the parent is not contributing, the treatment process takes longer. Many clients also want to see changes in their children right away and it is my job to explain to them that the child's symptoms or behaviors will not improve right away and the importance of their contribution to the child's treatment. Keeping my youth involved and engaged in therapy sessions has also been difficult.

One of my biggest struggles with TMH has been privacy. This has been a struggle because many of my clients will confirm being alone and in a private location, and then have side conversations in the middle of our session. Having those distractions has made it even more difficult for my clients to engage in our sessions. Building rapport is not an easy process when you do not have direct contact with the client, especially clients I begun seeing right before the pandemic and those I began with during TMH. Communication through TMH is something else I have struggled with. Many times, there are problems with the connection, and I have difficulty hearing my client or vice versa. Something unique about working with this population through TMH is that they are more likely to answer a phone call than they are to go to the clinic. Prior to this pandemic, there was at least one client each week that did not go to the clinic for their session. This made it difficult for me to gain my direct contact hours for my internship. Since doing TMH, almost all of my clients answer the phone every week.

For anyone that is interested in TMH, one piece of advice that I can give you is to be patient and open. There are many different tasks when doing TMH that you may not have had when doing in-person therapy. It is important for you to be patient with your clients, and also be prepared for the possibility that treatment through TMH will take a bit longer than in-person treatment may take. I think it is important for you to be open to things not going exactly as they would during in-person therapy.

REHABILITATION COUNSELING/CLINICAL REHABILITATION COUNSELING

Rehabilitation counselors "assist persons with physical, mental, developmental, cognitive, and emotional disabilities to achieve their personal, career, and independent living goals" (Commission on Rehabilitation Counselor Certification [CRCC], 2018, p. 2). Rehabilitation counselors provide counseling and related services to their clients including "communication, goal setting, and beneficial growth or change through self-advocacy, psychological, vocational, social, and behavioral interventions" (CRCC, 2018, p. 2). While other rehabilitation functions such as vocational evaluation, job development, case management, and work adjustment are related to the field of rehabilitation and may be included in a rehabilitation counselor's role, counseling remains the primary function of the rehabilitation counselor. Other functions that rehabilitation counselors may conduct include assessment, treatment planning, career counseling, group and individual counseling, service coordination, program evaluation, consultation, and assistance with accommodations (CRCC, 2018). While no state-level license for rehabilitation counselors currently exists, many counselors elect to earn their certified rehabilitation counselor (CRC) credential (CRCC, 2018). This is a national credential that may be a requirement for work in some positions, such as state-level vocational rehabilitation (VR) counselor positions.

CACREP currently accredits two rehabilitation counseling programs, Clinical Rehabilitation Counseling and Rehabilitation Counseling (CACREP, 2016). While both CACREP degree programs have a foundation in rehabilitation, clinical rehabilitation degrees include a foundation in biopsychosocial case conceptualization, treatment planning, neurological and biological foundations of disability, assessment, and screening. Conversely, rehabilitation counseling foundations include elements of vocational rehabilitation, self-determination, informed choice, societal inclusion, assessment, and accommodations (CACREP, 2016). Rehabilitation counseling programs were historically accredited by the Council on Rehabilitation Education (CORE), however, beginning in 2015, CACREP and CORE began a merger of the two organizations which was completed in 2017 (CACREP, 2020). Some universities offer a dual degree in clinical mental health counseling and clinical rehabilitation counseling, which resulted from the merger agreement. For simplicity, the term "rehabilitation counselor/counseling" will be utilized to encompass both rehabilitation counseling and clinical rehabilitation counseling specialties, unless otherwise noted.

The Centers for Disease Control and Prevention (CDC) describes a disability as the "absence of or significant difference in a person's body structure or function or mental functioning" (CDC, 2019, para. 6). A disability may be considered an impairment, activity limitation, or participation restriction. Disabilities may be a condition from birth, a result of a developmental condition, a result of an injury or accident, or a chronic illness including longstanding, progressive disorders. Disabilities may include sensory disorders, such as those impacting speech, vision, or hearing; cognitive disorders, including those impacting thinking, learning, or remembering; physical disabilities, including, mobility or health impairments; and social/emotional disorders including those that impact mental health, emotional responses, and social relationships (CDC, 2019). The Department of Education defines a person with a disability (PWD) as having "a physical or mental impairment that substantially limits a major life activity; has a record of such an impairment; or is regarded as having such an impairment" and notes that PWD have a long history of discriminatory harassment in the United States (U.S. Department of Education, 2020, para. 4). Federal laws such as the Individuals with Disabilities Act, the Rehabilitation Act, and the Americans with Disabilities Act mandate that PWD have equal access to opportunities, including education, employment, housing, and transportation.

Disability encompasses a broad spectrum of people, and PWD will seek services from rehabilitation counselors for a variety of needs, including vocational, social/emotional, living, and access issues. DC and TMH interventions are accommodations that rehabilitation counselors can utilize to assist PWD. Yet based on the varied and unique needs of the clients they serve, rehabilitation counselors will need to consider accessibility options and elements in their decision to use DC/TMH with their clients.

Evidence-Based Distance Counseling/Telemental Health Interventions in Rehabilitation Counseling

Research on the use of DC/TMH interventions in rehabilitation counseling spans the wide range of services that PWD may seek. Research tends to be clustered around three primary themes. First, vocational rehabilitation literature focuses on the use of technology to assist PWD with vocational goals and aspirations. This includes the growing area of assistive technology (AT). Assistive technology includes "equipment, or product system, whether acquired commercially off the shelf, modified, or customized, that is used to increase, maintain, or improve the functional capabilities" (U.S. Department of Education, 2017, para. 1). AT does not include medical devices, either external or implanted. A second body of literature focuses on clinical rehabilitation, such as using DC/TMH with PWD in relation to their mental health needs, as opposed to vocational needs. Finally, literature focuses on medical conditions and the use of DC/TMH interventions to improve emotional or personal functioning of persons with chronic medical conditions.

Vocational Rehabilitation

Research on the use of technology in vocational rehabilitation varies by the type of disability and person served. Individuals with traumatic brain injury (TBI) struggle with obtaining and maintaining employment. Due to physical, emotional, and cognitive symptoms, persons with TBI may struggle to organize and execute their job search, focus their attention while on the job, or interact socially with peers during interviews or work. Changes in routine or forgetfulness may impact job performance (Rumrill et al., 2016). Project Career is a multi-university initiative that involves referrals from university offices of disability support services, career services, and veteran student services. Students with TBI are provided with a series of assessments and then provided with an iPad specifically designed to support and train the students in areas of need such as memory, socialization, or other areas personalized to their symptoms and needs. These devices are also used for individual DC/TMH counseling. Individuals are encouraged to transfer these devices and learning tools to their work environment. One of the benefits of this model is that more and more individuals use iPads and devices in their daily functioning, so the iPad becomes more of a natural support than an accommodation for the PWD (Rumrill et al., 2016). Results of Project Career indicate that these technological interventions supported the majority of participants' academic success and transition to employment (Leopold et al., 2019).

Working with clients on the job site may be one element of vocational rehabilitation. In some agencies, job coaches or support specialists provide support to clients on the job, helping them learn their work role and appropriate interactions with staff. The use of technology, and specifically the use of videos, video prompts, audio files, and digital images, have been successfully used to support clients in learning jobs and related tasks. Specifically, clients with autism spectrum disorder (ASD) used mobile devices and audio/video image prompts to assist in learning their work roles. While some clients had greater success with the devices than others, the devices provided an option for reduced job coach contact and fostered independence among the clients (English et al., 2017; Van Laarhoven et al., 2019). The common use of iPads and other AT devices particularly among people with ASD and TBI is encouraging, since earlier evaluations indicated that AT was used primarily by persons with sensory and physical disorders, and rarely by those with cognitive or mental health disabilities (Huang et al., 2016).

Clinical Rehabilitation

Clinical rehabilitation counselors provide supports to clients in relation to their disability, as well as their mental health and emotional wellness. For example, deaf individuals may have difficulty accessing mental health treatment and counseling due to potential barriers in communication. Individuals who use American Sign Language (ASL) as their primary language, received education on TMH and a majority felt that TMH could benefit a variety of clinical needs. However, the most significant factor in whether the deaf person would use TMH was if they were unable to obtain counseling elsewhere (Crowe, 2017), which may indicate a preference for F2F services when available. One population that may struggle to seek services on their own are persons with severe and persistent mental illness (SPMI). Technical interventions have been utilized with this population with mixed results. Use of a medication management app, with telephone motivational interviewing sessions, were effective in reducing patient emergency department visits and maintaining medication compliance (Cook et al., 2008). However, the addition of an interactive, web-based program, in addition to in-person weekly recovery management sessions, did not consistently improve outcomes among those who participated in the web-based program (Beentjes et al., 2018).

Medical Conditions

Chronic medical conditions may lead to emotional distress. DC/TMH interventions have been used with patients experiencing symptoms such as depression and anxiety. Specifically, DC/TMH interventions have been successfully used with cancer patients (Bisseling et al., 2019), multiple sclerosis (Moss-Morris et al., 2012), irritable bowel syndrome (Andersson et al., 2011), and heart disease (Glozier et al., 2013; Lin et al., 2018). In these studies, various TMH interventions were utilized including self-help methods, group videoconference counseling, and iCBT interventions, both with and without therapist intervention. Indicators of success also varied in each study but included comparisons to F2F treatment, therapeutic alliance, and improved health, as well as reductions in depressive symptoms, each with favorable outcomes.

Ethical Issues in Rehabilitation Counseling and Distance Counseling/ Telemental Health

The American Rehabilitation Counseling Association (ARCA) is a chartered division of the ACA for rehabilitation counselors. The focus of ARCA is to support people with disabilities by encouraging ethical, effective, and efficient treatment among rehabilitation counselors. As a division of the ACA, ARCA members adhere to the ACA Code of Ethics. As has been discussed, the ACA Code of Ethics outlines in Section H detailed guidelines for professional counselors engaging in DC/TMH practices. While those guidelines will not be repeated here, it is important to note that professional counselors who are members of ARCA are expected to adhere to ACA Section H standards, as well as other elements of the code. As discussed, many rehabilitation counselors pursue the CRC certification, which is managed by the CRCC. The CRCC publishes the Code of Professional Ethics for Rehabilitation Counselors (2016), which includes ethical standards for the entirety of the rehabilitation counseling profession. Like other counseling organizations, the CRCC codes specify the unique needs of DC/TMH practice in a distinct section, namely Section J: Technology, Social Media, and Distance Counseling.

Rehabilitation counselors are expected to have the same level of competence in DC/TMH services as they provide in person (J1a). The CRCC requires rehabilitation counselors to adhere to all laws pertaining to DC/TMH in their own state, their clients' state, and international laws, as well as laws pertaining to digital confidentiality and security (J1b). Rehabilitation counselors must ensure that the technology they use is accessible for their clients, must assess if the technology is appropriate for the clients' needs (J2a), and must be sure that their clients have access to the technology (J2b). According to the CRCC, "clients have the freedom to choose whether to use technology-based distance counseling within the rehabilitation counseling process" (CRCC, 2016, p. 31), implying that counselors must be prepared to offer in-person services or refer those who do not wish to receive DC. The CRCC outlines several items to be included in the technology informed consent document, including risks and benefits of technology, plans for technology failure, anticipated response times, plans for when the counselor is not available, plans for emergencies, cultural or language differences, possible denial of insurance claims, social media policies, and more (J3a). Rehab counselors also discuss the risks of sending information via technology, such as email or text, with clients (J3b).

The CRCC requires that rehabilitation counselors utilize secure and encrypted technology (J3c), and also verify client identity during DC/TMH interactions (J3c). Rehabilitation counselors are required to have separate personal and professional social media accounts (J4a), and are expected to monitor their own social media activity to avoid, correct, or remove any content that could be harmful (J4b). Additionally, "rehabilitation counselors work within their organizations to develop and clearly communicate a social media policy so the social media practice is transparent, consistent, and easily understood by clients" (CRCC, 2016, p. 32). Counselors discuss the boundaries of social media (J4c), while also respecting the client's own privacy on social media. Rehabilitation counselors avoid searching a client's virtual presence "unless relevant to the rehabilitation counseling process" (J4d; CRCC, 2016, p. 32). Finally, rehabilitation counselors must avoid posting any personally identifying information without client permission (J4e). Because many rehabilitation counselors focus their work on employment and other goals, discussions about social media and online presence are a critical component of a client's presentation, professionalism, and self-advocacy.

The history of discrimination against PWD necessitates a need to address another area of the CRCC codes, specifically, Section C: Advocacy and Accessibility. Counselors from all specializations advocate for their clients and students, whether in a school, career, college, mental health or other counseling capacity. However due to the fact that PWD have historically been denied access to many rights and privileges, the rehabilitation counselor has added responsibilities in relation to advocacy and accessibility. In relation to technology used for DC/TMH interventions, PWD have unique access needs and may be subject to implicit biases that individuals without disabilities do not experience. Counselors may assume that DC/TMH intervention are preferred or convenient without clarifying the need or desire for DC/TMH services with the client. CRCC specifies "rehabilitation counselors address attitudinal barriers that inhibit the growth and development of their clients" (C1a) (CRCC, 2016, p.12). One example of an attitudinal barrier may be making decisions or assumptions on behalf of clients, without their desire or approval. For clients who do prefer DC/TMH interventions, rehabilitation counselors have a responsibility to facilitate reasonable accommodations in relation to services, programing, facilities, and technology (C2a). Additionally, they have a responsibility to make referrals only to resources that provide equitable accommodations (C2b), and to work with clients to develop strategies to address or eliminate barriers to access (C2c). Elements of Universal Design for Learning can serve as benchmarks for vocational rehabilitation services and referrals.

CASE STUDY: REHABILITATION COUNSELING

Counselor A is a vocational counselor who provides employment counseling and job placement services to adults receiving state vocational rehabilitation (VR) services. Counselor A is employed by a nonprofit agency that is contracted to provide VR services. Counselor A has been working with Client B who receives services for employment counseling and job placement. Client B is a 21-year-old individual with a diagnosis of cerebral palsy who uses an electric wheelchair for mobility. Client B has expressed an interest in a clerical position. Client B has good knowledge and experience with computers and technology, yet has fine motor limitations and mild speech delay. In addition to working with the vocational counselor,

Client B is also working with the housing counselor to obtain independent housing. Client B is motivated to work in order to supplement their income, which is needed to secure housing. Client B uses the public bus system for transportation or a shared van ride service. They prefer to use the bus because it is more affordable; however, Client B has shared that sometimes the bus driver does not know how to use the wheelchair lift, or the lift is not functional. Client B then needs to wait for the next bus, which often makes Client B late for appointments.

Counselor A would like to explore distance counseling sessions with Client B in order to reduce the cost and frustration of Client B's attending appointments at the office. Counselor A believes this will be a great way to continue to meet Client B, and also help them save money. Counselor A's agency does not provide distance counseling services, however the laptop that Counselor A is issued has a webcam, and Counselor A knows that they can get a free subscription to a videoconferencing program. Counselor A does not believe that Client B has access to a laptop, and asks the housing counselor if the agency had any loaners. The housing counselor suggests that Counselor A talk to the assistive technology (AT) specialist. Counselor A explains the situation to the AT specialist and is able to obtain a loaner laptop to provide to Client B. At their next meeting, Counselor A presents the laptop to Client B and explains that from now on, Counselor B does not need to come to the office and they can conduct all of their sessions via videoconferencing. Much to Counselor A's surprise, Client B does not seem happy about this arrangement and asks why they have to meet via videoconferencing instead of at the office.

DISCUSSION QUESTIONS

1. Consider Counselor A's training and preparation for DC. What did they do well and what could have been improved? What ethical concerns do you have?

2. Counselor A appears to have made some assumptions about Client B's preferences. What assumptions do you feel were made and what is the danger/risk in doing so?

3. How well suited do you feel Client B is for DC? What accommodations might be needed and how would you begin exploring those needs?

4. Consider Client B's perspective. What types of discrimination might they have experienced in the past? How might those experiences have impacted their response to Counselor A?

5. Assuming good intent, what did Counselor A do well?

CRITICAL QUESTIONS IN DECIDING TO PRACTICE

Rehabilitation counselors serve clients from diverse backgrounds, with unique needs. As such, rehabilitation counselors considering DC/TMH need to explore a variety of possibilities before implementing technological interventions.

1. What is your rehabilitation counseling role? Do you provide vocational rehabilitation counseling, clinical rehabilitation counseling, or other services?

2. What is the population of clients you serve and would DC be a benefit? How would you assess their developmental cognitive, cultural, and socioeconomic ability to use DC?

3. As always, what training do you have in DC/TMH counseling before expanding your practice to distance modalities?

4. As always, what TMH modalities will you use to offer treatment? How appropriate would various technologies be for the clients you serve, for example, phone, text, video?

5. Beyond encryption and HIPAA compliance, how is the technology you will use accessible to diverse populations? What accommodations would you need to make in order to best serve your clients?

6. What is your experience with AT? How knowledgeable are you on AT options that your clients might need/consider?

7. PWD have experienced a history of discrimination in the United States. How might you explore these issues with your clients, while also monitoring your own biases? How can the use of technology help/hinder this process?

8. PWD encounter assumptions and implicit biases on a daily basis. How might you explore these issues with your clients, while also monitoring your own assumptions? How can the use of technology help/hinder this process?

9. Rehabilitation counselors have a professional responsibility to advocate for their clients. How can technology beyond the use of DC/TMH be used in client advocacy?

10. Consider the CRCC Code of Ethics in its entirety. How well does your practice adhere to them?

VOICES FROM THE FIELD

Vocational Rehabilitation Using Videoconferencing

Heather C. Robertson, PhD, CRC, LMHC, GCDF, BC-TMH

I serve as a part-time, fee-for-service vocational rehabilitation counselor for an agency, in addition to my full-time role as a counselor educator. I provide vocational rehabilitation (VR) counseling to adults receiving state VR services and high school special education students preparing for school-to-work transitions. I provided distance counseling via secure videoconferencing to some of my clients prior to the COVID-19 closures, and all of my clients post-COVID-19. I've had the benefit of being able to see my same clients both in person and online, which I know is not feasible for all counselors.

The benefit of DC in a VR setting is the ability to meet the client where they are at, both literally and figuratively. For clients who need to utilize a shared-van ride service (which is not great in my area), the ability to eliminate that cost or frustration for them, even once, demonstrates empathy and understanding. Also, because of the wide variety of career resources online (e.g., labor market information, career assessments, digital portfolios, online job searches), the use of a "share screen" feature allows me to help the client navigate these systems. I've also had clients who, depending on their diagnosis, struggle to make appointments or leave the house. In these cases, DC allows me to meet with the client, as opposed to them canceling or no-showing. Conversely, since my role is to prepare clients for the world of work, I do need to ultimately help them leave their house and be on time for appointments. This point leads me to offer the following cautions when using DC in VR.

I find that the success of the DC depends on both the client's overall functioning and their ability to utilize the technology. With my high school students, such as those with Autism Spectrum Disorders, I'm pretty sure they prefer meeting online to meeting in person. They can navigate the computer or tablet with ease, and seem to adapt seamlessly to our online sessions. For other clients, I found the distance sessions to be less effective. For some clients with mental health disorders, when I met these clients in the office, they would prepare by showering, dressing, and bringing materials for our meeting. Online, the lack of structure and/or the comfort of their home, was less suitable to our work. Despite my instructions, some clients were unprepared to work during online sessions. Some days they used their phone, which was challenging to see career information on screen. In one case, I stopped video sessions with a client because they were not productive. I actually felt uncomfortable billing for sessions where we spent half the time navigating technology or waiting for the client to get dressed.

My advice to rehabilitation counselors considering distance counseling would be to ensure that your agency has the proper technology and training to conduct distance sessions. It's important to discuss the expectations of these distance sessions with your clients, as well as parents if you are working with minors. Finally, if you find that distance services are not effective, don't be afraid to revert back to in-person sessions, if that is an option.

CONCLUSION

All individuals in life experience transition and may seek help from professional counselors. Marriage, couple, and family counselors have successfully used DC/TMH with military families, parent and child relationships, as well as couples counseling. The IAMFC publishes a professional code of ethics for marriage, couple, and family counselors, yet also specifies that these codes are designed to supplement codes provided by the ACA. Like other professional organizations, the IAMFC specifies ethical practice pertaining to DC/TMH through Section I: Technology Assisted Couples and Family Counseling. Rehabilitation counselors assist individuals with disabilities on their personal, social, emotional, and vocational goals. Many rehabilitation counselors earn their CRC credential. PWD have benefited from DC/TM interventions. Research in the areas of vocational rehabilitation, clinical rehabilitation, and medical conditions have found that, overall, DC/TMH interventions benefit PWD. The ARCA is a chartered division of the ACA for rehabilitation counselors. While ARCA does not publish their own ethical codes, they also require adherence to the ACA Code of Ethics. The CRCC publishes ethical codes for rehabilitation counselors, and specific DC/TMH content in Section J: Technology, Social Media, and Distance Counseling. PWD have a history of discrimination in the United States and rehabilitation counselors must also recognize their responsibility to advocate and promote accessibility for their clients.

REFERENCES

American Counseling Association. (2014). *2014 ACA code of ethics.* https://www .counseling.org/Resources/aca-code-of-ethics.pdf

Anderson, K. E., Byrne, C. E., Crosby, R. D., & Le Grange, D. (2017). Utilizing telehealth to deliver family-based treatment for adolescent anorexia nervosa. *International Journal of Eating Disorders, 50,* 1235–1238. https://doi.org/10.1002/ eat.22759

Andersson, E., Ljótsson, B., Smit, F., Paxling, B., Hedman, E., Lindefors, N., Andersson, G., & Rück, C. (2011). Cost-effectiveness of internet-based cognitive behavior therapy for irritable bowel syndrome: results from a randomized controlled trial. *BMC Public Health, 11,* 215–222. https://doi.org/10.1186/1471-2458-11-215

Beentjes, T. A. A., Goosens, P. J. J., Vermeulen, H., Teerenstra, S., Nijuis-van der Sanden, M. W. G., & van Gaal, B. I. G. (2018). E-IMR: e-health added to face-to-face delivery of Illness Management & Recovery programme for people with severe mental illness, an exploratory clustered randomized controlled trial. *BMC Health Services Research, 18,* 962. https://doi.org/10.1186/s12913-018-3767-5

Bisseling, E., Cillessen, L., Spinhoven, P., Schellekens, M., Compen, F., van der Lee, M., & Speckens, A. (2019). Development of therapeutic alliance and its association with treatment outcome in internet based Mindfulness-Based Cognitive Therapy (eMBCT) compared to group-based MBCT (MBCT) for distressed cancer patients. *Journal of Psychosomatic Research, 121,* 146–147. https://doi.org/10.1016/j.jpsychores.2019.03.141

Blom, M. M., Bosmans, J. E., Cuijpers, P., Zarit, S. H., & Pot, A. M. (2013). Effectiveness and cost-effectiveness of an internet intervention for family caregivers of people with dementia: design of a randomized controlled trial. *BMC Psychiatry, 13,* 1–7. http://www.biomedcentral.com/1471-244X/13/17

Center for Disease Control and Prevention. (2019). *Disability and health overview.* https://www.cdc.gov/ncbddd/disabilityandhealth/disability.html

Cicila, L. N., Georgia, E., J., & Doss, B. D. (2014). Incorporating internet-based interventions into couple therapy: Available resources and recommended uses. *The Australian & New Zealand Journal of Family Therapy, 35,* 414–430. https://doi.org/10.1002/anzf.1077

Comer, J. S., Furr, J. M., Miguel, E. M., Cooper-Vince, C. E., Carpenter, A. L., Elkins, R. M., Kerns, C. E., Cornacchio, D., Chou, T., Coxe, S., DeSerisy, M., Sanchez, A. L., . . . Chase, R. (2017). Remotely delivering real-time parent training to the home: An initial randomized trial of Internet-Delivered Child-Parent Interaction Therapy (I-PCIT). *Journal of Consulting and Clinical Psychology, 86,* 909–917. https://doi.org/10.1037/ccp0000230

Commission on Rehabilitation Counselor Certification. (2016). *Code of professional ethics for rehabilitation counselors.* https://www.crccertification.com/filebin/Ethics_Resources/CRCC_Code_Eff_20170101.pdf

Commission on Rehabilitation Counselor Certification. (2018). *Career series promote your credential: Rehabilitation Counseling scope of practice.* https://www.crccertification.com/filebin/pdf/careercenter/CRCC_ScopeOfPractice.pdf

Cook, P. F., Emiliozzi, S., Waters, C., & El Haji, D. (2008). Effects of telephone counseling on antipsychotic adherence and emergency department utilization. *The American Journal of Managed Care, 14,* 841–846.

Council on the Accreditation of Counseling and Related Education Programs. (2016). *2016 CACREP Standards and Glossary.* http://www.cacrep.org/wp-content/uploads/2018/05/2016-Standards-with-Glossary-5.3.2018.pdf

Council on the Accreditation of Counseling and Related Education Programs. (2020). *CACREP/CORE Merger Information.* https://www.cacrep.org/home/cacrepcore-updates

Crowe, T. V. (2017). Is telemental health services a viable alternative to traditional psychotherapy for deaf individuals? *Community Mental Health Journal, 53,* 154–162. https://doi.org/10.1007/s10597-016-0025-3

Doss, B. D., Feinberg, L. K., Rothman, K., Roddy, M. K., & Comer, J. S. (2017). Using technology to enhance and expand interventions for couples and families: Conceptual and methodological considerations. *Journal of Family Psychology, 31,* 983–993. https://doi.org/10.1037/fam0000349

English, D. L., Gounden, S., Dagher, R. E., Chan, S. F, Furlonger, B. E., Anderson, A., & Moore, D. W. (2017). Effects of video modeling with video feedback on vocational skills of adults with autism spectrum disorder. *Developmental Neurohabilitation, 20,* 511–524. https://doi.org/10.1080/17518423.2017.1282051

Glozier, N., Christensen, H., Naismith, S., Cockayne, N., Donkin, L., Neal, B., Mackinnon, A., & Hickie, I. (2013). Internet-delivered cognitive behavioural therapy for adults with mild to moderate depression and high cardiovascular disease risks: A randomised attention-controlled trial. *PLoS ONE, 8*(3), 1–8. https://doi.org/10.1371/journal.pone.0059139

Huang, I-C., Chieng, G., Rumrill, P., Bengston, K., Chan, F., Telzlaff, J., & Snitker, M. (2016). Characteristics of people with disabilities receiving assistive technology services in vocational rehabilitation: A logistical regression analysis. *Journal of Vocational Rehabilitation 45,* 63–72. https://doi.org/10.3233/JVR-160811

International Association of Marriage and Family Counselors. (2017). *IAMFC Code of Ethics.* https://www.iamfconline.org/public/IAMFC-Ethical-Code-Final.pdf

Kersting, A., Kroker, K., Schlicht, S., Baust, K., & Wagner, B. (2011). Efficacy of cognitive-behavioral internet-based therapy in parents after loss of child during pregnancy: Pilot data from randomized controlled trial. *Archive of Women's Health, 14,* 465–477. https://doi.org/10.1007/s00737-011-0240-4

Leopold, A., Rumrill, P., Hendricks, D. J., Nardone, A., Sampson, E., Minton, D., Jacobs, K., Elias, E., & Scherer, M. (2019). A mixed-methodological examination of participant experiences, activities, and outcomes in a technology and employment project for postsecondary students with traumatic brain injury. *Journal of Vocational Rehabilitation, 50,* 3–11. https://doi.org/10.3233/JVR-180983

Lin, T., Yu, P., Lin, L., Liu, P., Li, Y., Hsu, C., Cheng, Y., Yeh, C., Wong, S., Pai, S., Shee, H., & Weng, C. (2018). A pilot-study to assess the feasibility and acceptability of an Internet-based cognitive-behavior group therapy using video conference for patients with coronary artery heart disease. *PLoS ONE, 13*(11), 1–13. https://doi.org/10.1371/journal.pone.0207931

Mogil, C., Hajal, N., Garcia, E., Kiff, C., Paley, B., Milburn, N., & Lester, P. (2015). FOCUS for early childhood: A virtual home visiting program for military families with young children. *Contemporary Family Therapy, 37,* 199–208. https://doi.org/10.1007/s10591-015-9327-9

Moss-Morris, R., McCrone, P., Yardley, L., van Kessel, K., Wills, G., & Dennison, L. (2012). A pilot randomised controlled trial of an Internet-based cognitive behavioural therapy self-management programme (MS Invigor8) for multiple sclerosis fatigue. *Behaviour Research & Therapy, 50,* 415–422. https://doi.org/10.1016/j.brat.2012.03.001

Palermo, T. M., Law, E. F., Fales, J., Bromberg, M. H., Jessen-Fiddick, T., & Tai, G. (2016). Internet-delivered cognitive-behavioral treatment for adolescents with chronic pain and their parents: A randomized controlled multicenter trial. *Pain, 157,* 174-185. https://doi.org/10.1097/j.pain.0000000000000348

Price, L. E., Noulas, P., Wen, I., & Spray, A. (2018). A portal to healing: Treating military families and veterans through telehealth. *Journal of Clinical Psychology, 75,* 271–281. https://doi.org/10.1002/jclp.22720

Rumrill, P., Elias, E., Hendricks, D. J., Jacobs, K., Leopold, A., Nardone, A., Sampson, E., Scherer, M., Stauffer, C., & McMahon, B. T. (2016). Promoting cognitive support technology use and employment success among post-secondary students with traumatic brain injury. *Journal of Vocational Rehabilitation, 45,* 53–61. https://doi.org/10.3233/JVR-160810

Schlossberg, N. K. (2011). The challenge of change: The transition model and its application. *Journal of Employment Counseling, 48,* 159–162. https://doi.org/10.1002/j.2161-1920.2011.tb01102.x

Van Laarhoven, T., Carreon, A., Bonneau, W., & Lagerhausen, A. (2018). Comparing mobile technologies for teaching vocational skills to individuals with Autism Spectrum Disorders and/or intellectual disabilities using universally-designed prompting systems. *Journal of Autism and Developmental Disorders, 48,* 2516–2529. https://doi.org/10.1007/s10803-018-3512-2

U.S. Department of Education. (2017). *Individuals with Disabilities Education Act. Sec. 300.5.* Assistive technology. https://sites.ed.gov/idea/regs/b/a/300.5

U.S. Department of Education. (2020). *Office of Civil Rights.* Disability Discrimination. https://www2.ed.gov/about/offices/list/ocr/frontpage/faq/disability.html

12

The Future of Distance Counseling and Telemental Health

INTRODUCTION

Distance counseling (DC)/telemental health (TMH) is here, and here to stay. It's not the future and not "coming soon." It's not a stop-gap measure in the wake of COVID-19. It has arrived, and was already well-integrated into the profession of counseling prior to the COVID-19 crisis. Despite its arrival and infiltration, DC/TMH interventions will evolve. The profession and the public continue to become more accustomed to DC/TMH interventions, as they do other distance services, including working from home and conducting appointments virtually, such as medical appointments. Following COVID-19, it is yet to be determined how the world will maintain its distance practices, or if there will be a return to more "traditional," face-to-face (F2F) interactions that were utilized prior to the pandemic.

There is ample evidence that the COVID-19 crisis will have a long-standing impact on our nation's economy and individual well-being. Global deaths resulting from COVID-19 number in the hundreds of thousands, with a significant portion of those deaths being recorded in the United States (World Health Organization [WHO], 2020). A disproportionate number of U.S. COVID-19 deaths and infections are recorded among

Black and Hispanic communities (Centers for Disease Control and Prevention [CDC], 2020). In April of 2020, the Bureau of Labor Statistics (BLS) reported that unemployment rose 10% increasing to 14.7%, the result of the loss of 20.5 million nonfarm jobs in the United States during the month of April (BLS, 2020). Like the COVID-19 deaths and illness, these unemployment rates are not distributed equitably, with greater rates of unemployment among Black and Hispanic populations (BLS, 2020). Parents of school-aged children who maintained their jobs are struggling to manage work-from-home and home-schooling responsibilities simultaneously. There are indications that stay-at-home orders increased the probability of domestic violence, substance use relapse, and child abuse (New York State Office of Mental Health, 2020), particularly as children are out of school where abuse may be observed or reported. In the midst of these crises, or perhaps because of them, people are experiencing grief, loss, depression, anxiety, anger, frustration, and other emotions that impact their well-being. It is clear that the need for professional counseling for children and adults will persist long after the COVID-19 crisis passes. However, the delivery of counseling will likely look drastically different than it had prior to, or even in the midst of, this crisis.

PURSUING CERTIFICATION IN TELEMENTAL HEALTH COUNSELING

The need for counselor training in DC/TMH prior to engaging in practice has been included in nearly every counseling ethical code addressed throughout this book. Some might argue that receiving any training is sufficient for DC/TMH practice. Conversely, this book has addressed the wide variation in TMH training programs, including differences in content, hours, and cost. Professional counselors are left with little direction on how and which training program to select. Most likely, the public consumer is unaware of these training variations, and may not know if their DC/TMH-trained counselor had 5 hours of training or 500 hours. Finally, state laws vary on requirements to provide TMH services, while some specializations, such as career counseling, are not regulated by state licensure boards. Insurance companies may also have different requirements for DC/TMH providers on their panels. One way to standardize these variations in training is to offer a certificate or credential that meets unified standards.

The process of credentialing and certification has multiple purposes. First, it provides legitimacy to the practice, and sets a standard for training and/or experience. Second, it serves to protect the public from the potential harm of incompetence or untrained individuals. However, "some credentials are essential to the practice of the profession, others are desirable but not necessary, and still others are of questionable value or even worthless" (Remley & Herlihy, 2016, p. 33). The public and the profession, as well as state licensing boards and insurance companies, will have to determine if certification in DC/TMH couseling is essential, desirable, questionable, or worthless. Based on the nuances of DC/TMH discussed throughout this book and the potential for risk and liability, it can be argued that certification is necessary in order to ensure counselor competence and to protect client safety. Despite this argument, it is yet to be seen if DC/TMH certification will be adopted broadly, or if clinicians will continue the learn-as-you-go model that was utilized by many during COVID-19.

Gaining broad acceptance of a credential or standard across the counseling profession will not be accomplished easily. The American Counseling Association (ACA) embarked on an initiative known as *20/20: A Vision for the Future of Counseling*. Beginning in 2005, the ACA and representatives from 30 professional counseling organizations came together to develop a standard definition, title, and educational foundation for professional counselors (Gerig, 2018) by the year 2020. While the group was successful in developing a unified title and definition of professional counseling, the group could not reach consensus on educational requirements. It is feasible to imagine this process repeating itself as counselors struggle with the concept of unified training and credentialing for DC/TMH interventions.

The Board-Certified Telemental Health provider (BC-TMH) is a national credential offered by the Center for Credentialing in Education (CCE, 2020), which is an affiliate of the National Board of Certified Counselors (NBCC). Currently this credential is available to a wide variety of professional licenses and certifications, with completion of an approved training program, passing of a standard exam, and applying/paying for the credential. BC-TMH providers must also complete continuing education in order to maintain their credential. The BC-TMH extends far beyond professional counseling to include areas such as registered nurses, physician assistants, and other helping professions, among them marriage and family therapists, psychologists, and social workers. Interestingly, there is no approved BC-TMH credential for career counselors, despite the fact that a variety of career counselors deliver DC services. In addition, there is no provision for state-certified school counselors to earn the BC-TMH, although Nationally Certified School Counselors (NCSC) and Nationally Certified Counselors (NCC) may apply for the credential. Unintentionally, the title of the certification, with its emphasis on telemental health counseling, may dissuade those whose professional identity does not include mental health counseling from applying, including school counselors, career counselors, and student affairs counselors. For the school, career, and student affairs professionals who plan to practice distance counseling, which certification or training should they complete, if any?

This question and others will need to be addressed in the future, as the use of DC/TMH becomes mainstream in counseling practice. Will the counseling profession—as a whole—adopt a standard credential for telemental health, such as the BC-TMH? Will the profession continue to separate or exempt the work of nonclinical counselors from DC/TMH certification and training, despite awareness that they engage in distance practice? Will the profession adapt current training and certification processes to be inclusive of these nonclinical specializations? Will states require some sort of certification or training to practice DC/TMH, and will that requirement be a national standard or a state-by-state determination? These questions are reminiscent of supervisor credentialing within the counseling profession. The CCE also offers the Approved Clinical Supervisor (ACS) credential, which, similar to the BC-TMH, requires a mental health degree and mental health experience. Like clinical mental health counselors, school counselors and career counselors also require supervision, but are unable to earn the ACS credential. Interestingly, the National Career Development Association's (NCDA) code of ethics requires training before engaging in DC practice, yet career counselors are unable to earn the BC-TMH because they lack a license or credential that is deemed appropriate for the BC-TMH. If credentialing for these specializations is not available for DC practice, the profession and the public are again left with the question of how much training is necessary, if any. While career counselors and others can elect to attend other training programs, the CCE's affiliation with NBCC provides an opportunity to promote a unified training standard and credential to all professional counselors via the BC-TMH or a similar credential.

PROFESSIONAL DEVELOPMENT IN TELEMENTAL HEALTH COUNSELING

Professional credentialing, while legitimizing the field and protecting clients, has the added benefit of helping counselors remain current through additional training and professional development. Technology moves at a rapid pace and technological advances change multiple times throughout one's life time. Consider the advances in medicine that are made over a decade due to technology; the medical provider who is not using these advances is missing an opportunity to help patients. As in DC/TMH counseling, the information that one receives in one's training in 2020 may no longer be valid in 2028, particularly with the rate at which technology changes. This is another argument for a professional credential in DC/TMH, such as the BC-TMH program, that requires counselors to obtain continuing education in order to maintain the credential. However, if the credential is not valued or required by state licensing boards, insurance companies, or the public, some practitioners will not elect to complete a voluntary credential. Thus, there will be no oversight as to whether these counselors elect to stay current in their professional development training. Clearly there are no easy answers to the issues of credentialing, training, and certification.

Professional development remains a critical component of the counseling profession, regardless of requirements and certifications. As new issues emerge and develop in counseling specialty areas, counselors need to remain abreast of these issues and learn how to best serve their clients and students in relation to this new information. While some counselors may decide not to remain current in the profession, minimally all professional counseling ethical codes require that counselors maintain current, evidence-based, best practices. The profession has already experienced how technology can provide opportunities for professional development. Live and recorded **webinars** allow counselors to learn from experts around the globe in a variety of specializations and issues. Similarly, **online education** allows counselors to complete courses, certificates, and academic degrees in synchronous or asynchronous formats. More recently, **virtual conferences** have emerged in which counselors can both present and attend a professional conference via the Internet. In addition to professional development, these training programs often offer **continuing education (CE)** hours that counselors can use to maintain their licenses and credentials. Some credentials may limit the amount of hours that can be completed online for the recredentialing process, although fewer agencies are following this practice in the aftermath of COVID-19.

Technologies have emerged that allow clients to enhance their skills, as opposed to simply earning CE hours. The concept of deliberate practice allows practitioners to use technology to practice basic and advanced counseling skills and interventions (Elliot et al., 2018; Fredrickson & Rousmaniere, 2018). Much like a musician or an athlete improves with practice, counselors who deliberately practice specific skills will improve upon those skills, and ultimately have better outcomes with the clients and students they serve (K. Shuster, personal communication, May 28, 2020). The challenge of practice in live counseling, however, is that counseling sessions do not allow the counselor to repeatedly practice the same skill over and over, nor do live counseling sessions allow counselors to specify which skill they wish to practice. The client should be directing the session, and the counselor is required to respond to whatever the client brings to session. Thus, deliberate practice uses technological platforms that include audio and/or video recordings and allow counselors to practice specific skills in relation to a client scenario. These deliberate practice recordings can then be reviewed by professors, supervisors, or peers for professional feedback. Because they are often recorded in response to actors in fabricated scenarios, there is less risk of confidentiality breaches. Some systems allow the user to complete a self-evaluation and re-record their practice sessions prior to submitting them to a reviewer (K. Shuster, personal communication, May 28, 2020).

The technology for professional development and practice sessions will continue to grow. There has been an emergence of training using **artificial intelligence (AI)** and avatars. These training and simulation programs have been used to help professionals learn to manage crisis situations that cannot be easily replicated in a role play or classroom simulation. The profession has also seen an emergence of **virtual reality (VR)** therapeutic interventions, such as virtual reality exposure therapy (Riva & Repetto, 2016). These advancements are making their way to counselor training, where future counselors-in-training can sit down with virtual clients and practice their skills in a setting that simulates realistic counseling scenarios. Just as technology is used to enhance the services provided to clients, technology can be utilized to enhance the training of professional counselors before they engage in practice.

A variety of DC/TMH resources are available for counselors to either remain current on their DC/TMH practice, or learn more about DC/TMH. As has been discussed, Epstein Becker Green Law (2017) publishes a 50-state guide to telemental health practice laws, which is now available as a mobile app for easy updates. The Zur Institute (2020), while designed as a paid continuing education resource, offers a variety of free resources to the public on telemental health including listings of Health Insurance Portability and Accountability Act (HIPAA) compliant software, state-by-state comparisons of telemental health terminology, a listing of the major telemental health ethical codes across a variety of professions, and many other resources. The American Telemedicine Association (ATA) is likely one of the largest interdisciplinary organizations focused on telemedicine, including telehealth. Membership includes medical providers and mental health providers, yet at the time of this publication, may be costly for an individual provider. While many resources are only available to members, there are a variety of free resources and articles available to the public (2020). The Online Therapy Institute also offers specialized training programs for working with children, coaching, or providing distance supervision (2020), but may require a fee.

The variety of ethical standards from counseling-specific professional organizations has been addressed throughout this book, including the American Counseling Association (ACA), the American School Counseling Association (ASCA), the American Mental Health Counselors Association (AMHCA), the National Career Development Association (NCDA), Commission for the Credentialing of Rehabilitation Counselors (CRCC), and other counseling organizations, as well as standards from organizations such as CAS and NAADAC. Each of these organizations, beyond their ethical standards, also post a variety of resources on their websites pertaining to DC/TMH and their counseling specialization. Similarly, federal organizations such as the Substance Abuse and Mental Health Services Administration (SAMHSA) publish guidelines and recommendations for telehealth (2020), while other organizations have posted resources specifically in response to COVID-19. These free and public resources provide opportunities for counselors to remain current and expand their knowledge of DC/TMH interventions.

BEGINNING A TELEMENTAL HEALTH PRACTICE

The choice of whether or not to begin a DC/TMH practice is an important decision. Many counselors may indeed have a "choice" as to whether or not they want to expand their practice to DC/TMH interventions. Those counselors are encouraged to weigh their decisions based on their ability to obtain and maintain many of the practice standards outlined in this book. However, in the wake of the COVID-19 pandemic, some counselors and counselor-interns had no choice; services were moved to online and distance formats and counselors were forced to adapt. Many graduate-level interns were faced with the challenge of not specifically wanting to engage in TMH before solidifying their F2F training, but also facing the reality of needing to earn enough direct counseling hours in order to graduate. Regardless of how one arrives at DC/TMH practice – either via choice or necessity – the onus of responsibility continues to fall on the professional counselor, as opposed to the agency or the client. Thus professional counselors are wise to engage in thoughtful reflection prior to engaging in DC/TMH practice. Those thrust into DC/TMH practice without preparation or reflection are encouraged to engage in this process immediately. The ability for a counselor to reflect, make decisions, and alter practices demonstrates a commitment to ethics and client well-being, and may serve as a mitigating factor for future liability and risk.

This book has outlined a variety of strategies pertaining to DC/TMH practice, as well as a variety of cautions. Foundational factors include receiving DC/TMH training, utilizing secure and encrypted technologies, determining if DC/TMH is appropriate for your clients/students, determining if your clients/students have access to technology, considering cultural implications, being aware of TMH laws in your area, and adhering to all professional ethical codes applicable to your specialization. Appendix 12.A includes a detailed checklist of the major elements from the book for counselors to review prior to practice. While some counselors view DC/TMH as an opportunity to expand their income and revenue, it is equally important to consider the cost and investment of establishing a quality practice. Counselors may underestimate the costs of equipment, administrative software, quality video camera technologies, training, and technical support (Zimmerman & Magnavita, 2018). Providing high-quality

DC/TMH services is an investment not only of financial means, but of one's time. The primary purpose of this book is to allow counselors an opportunity to reflect on the elements of DC/TMH practice before engaging in unethical, ineffective, or even dangerous treatment of clients. Beneficence and non-maleficence are guiding principles of every professional counseling role, and taking the time to prepare for DC/TMH interventions upholds these principles.

COUNSELOR SELF-CARE

One of the hallmarks of the counseling profession is being wellness-focused, and viewing client concerns from a wellness model (Gerig, 2018). Yet the demands of the counseling profession may put the counselor's own wellness at risk. To begin, one of the benefits of DC/TMH services is access. This has been mentioned by multiple practitioners in the "Voices From the Field" contributions that were received for this book. Providing DC/TMH helps clients access counselors and hopefully access the treatment that they might otherwise have not received. Yet with **increased access** may come increased demands. A client's ability to access a counselor via email, text, or telephone may **blur professional boundaries**. Counselors may feel obligated to respond to client inquiries immediately, as one would do if the client were sitting across from you in the office or sitting out in the waiting area. Many counselors pride themselves on being responsive to clients' needs. Second, the role of the professional counseling carries with it the risk of **burnout and vicarious trauma,** regardless of DC/TMH practice. A professional counselor repeatedly bears witness to the struggles and crises of their clients. The weight of these narratives run the risk of damaging the counselor who does not engage in wellness strategies, including their own supervision and counseling. Elements that may contribute to vicarious trauma include lack of experience, lack of supervision, and lack of trauma-related knowledge (Naghavi & Salimi, 2018). Finally, issues of **social justice and equity** continue to plague our society. As the world was attempting to rebound from the COVID-19 crisis, the deaths of Amaud Abrey, Breonna Taylor, and George Floyd again raised issues of police brutality and white privilege in the United States. Counselors, who are supposed to be focused on the needs of their clients and students, find themselves struggling with their own emotions—or those of their clients—and feelings of helplessness against injustice. The magnitude and scope of these issues are not easily packed away for an hour-long session, but continue to erode at a counselor's core energy if not addressed.

Professional boundaries and self-care are essential to maintaining a counselor's own wellness, which in turn preserves their ability to provide competent, quality care to the clients and students they serve. Counselors often encourage their clients to engage in self-care or mindfulness, but may fail to implement these strategies in their own lives. Self-care is an ethical mandate (ACA, 2014). Work-related stress often contributes to feelings of burnout, which is why it is critical to set a schedule and communication boundaries (Coaston, 2017) when working with clients remotely. The DC/TMH counselor should have a not-available contact plan, where clients know who they should be contacting, including emergency personnel, when the counselor is not available. Coaston (2017) advocates for a self-compassionate mindset, explaining that many wellness plans are too vague and allow opportunity for self-criticism. It is more helpful for the counselor to develop an awareness of their own signs of burnout and stress, and then seek to implement strategies to alleviate those symptoms by implementing interventions for the mind, body, and spirit. Technology can provide a variety of resources, through mobile apps, to assist the client with their overall self-compassion plan. Coaston (2017) also recommends intellectual stimulation, such as writing, journaling, blogging, or even keeping notes of positive memories and gratitude to combat the weight of absorbed client traumas.

The transition to DC/TM interventions following the COVID-19 stay-at-home orders was swift and sudden, and the impact of COVID-19 was significant. Many people were experiencing death, loss, grief, and unemployment, in addition to the issues of police brutality and white privilege already described. Counselors regularly step in to help people after crises, such as hurricanes, tornados, and other natural disasters. Yet in the case of COVID-19, the counselors themselves were experiencing the same traumas as the clients they were serving via DC/TMH interventions. In previous studies in which counselors experienced the same crises as their clients, counselors reported personal feelings of "emotional vulnerability, the challenge of loss, the new normal, and a different way of existing" (Cooper et al., 2018, p. 435). Ethically, volunteers felt a responsibility to help, but professionally felt as if they were "flying by the seat of their pants" (p. 436). Counselors were experiencing uncertainty, personal losses of their own, and similar experiences as the clients they were attempting to serve. In these circumstances, managing professional boundaries and allowing time away from the crisis area was recommended. Specialized training such as psychological first aid or disaster response training is necessary to assist counselors in managing client cases. Other protective factors to reduce vicarious trauma may include counseling, peer support, and gaining knowledge of trauma and crisis work (Naghavi & Salimi, 2018).

Self-care is also important for supervisees and counseling students. Counselor educators can implement instructional strategies for burnout and self-care. The use of a 1.5-hour psychoeducation session on burnout and weekly check-ins was determined to have assisted counselors-in-training with self-care, accountability, burnout awareness, and healthy coping strategies (Lindo et al., 2015). Other educators recommend teaching self-compassion to counselors-in-training, including self-kindness, common humanity, and mindfulness, as a component of their self-care strategy (Nelson et al., 2018). Finally, client advocacy is included in the role of a professional counselor (ACA, 2014). While some counselors may interpret this standard to mean individual client advocacy, counselors may also elect to take a larger role in advocacy issues in response to issues of social justice and inequity. It has been recommended that counselors become socially active, participate in social movements, and volunteer with professional organizations (Roysircar, 2009).

IMPLICATIONS FOR COUNSELOR EDUCATORS AND SUPERVISORS

Certification and training is one format of learning DC/TMH practice. The process of certification and training contains a variety of complexities, as discussed. Other ways of developing competence include educational degree programs, as well as supervision. For most counseling specialties discussed in this book, a master's degree is required. Supervision is required during field work in the graduate program, as well as in the post-master's program, for some specializations such as Clinical Mental Health Counseling.

This book has regularly referenced the Council on the Accreditation of Counseling and Related Education (CACREP) standards. It has been noted that CACREP standards require trainees to understand the impact of technology on the counseling process, but not specifically how to use technology in the counseling process (2016). Despite this shortcoming, the inclusion of technology content in the 2016 CACREP standards exceeded technology content included in the 2009 version (Sykes Stretch et al., 2016). Thus it is possible that the 2023 CACREP standards will further address DC/TMH interventions. Another organization, known as Masters in Psychology and Counseling Accreditation Council (MPCAC), also accredits master's level counseling and counseling psychology programs. MPCAC standards (2017) require knowledge and skills in areas such as ethics, theory, multiculturalism, and others. However, the standards fail to use the word technology at any point within the curricular standards. Master's programs continue to be the standard level of educational preparation for professional counselors, and the use of DC/TMH interventions continue to grow. As a result, counselor education programs will need to determine if learning to practice in DC/TMH modalities is foundational to master's-level learning.

The alternative to master's-level learning is to continue to view DC/TMH as a post-master's training option. Unfortunately, during COVID-19, many academic institutions had to rush to develop TMH training curricula, provide TMH training, develop contingency internship sites, or rely on internship sites to train students in DC/TMH. As already addressed, it is likely that in the post-COVID-19 era, DC/TMH interventions will be more common. Just as internship sites expect students to enter the site with foundational skills in counseling, they may soon expect interns to possess foundational skills in DC/TMH interventions upon entering the internship. Counseling program accrediting organizations, such as CACREP and MPCAC, will need to consider the inclusion of DC/TMH knowledge and content, as well as practice, into their curricular standards. Depending on the institution's instructional format, DC/TMH instructional content may vary. Just as online counseling programs teach F2F skills via a distance platform, in-person educational programs will need to find avenues to teach students how to counsel in a DC/TMH setting. More importantly, counselor education faculty will need to be prepared and qualified to teach DC/TMH to the next generation of counselors. Should accrediting organizations require training in DC/TMH interventions, counselor education programs may struggle to identify competent faculty to teach such content. This is particularly relevant for institutions that are unable to utilize adjunct or part-time faculty, indicating that the current faculty must already possess, or be willing to gain, the knowledge and competence to teach DC/TMH interventions to counselors-in-training.

Supervision of counselors is a critical component of counselor development. Counselors engage in supervision during graduate-level internships, and for some specializations, post-master's supervision is needed in order to earn a counseling license. Distance supervision, also referred to as cybersupervision (Coursol et al., 2016), can be utilized to provide supervision to counselors in a variety of settings, including rural communities, or those seeking supervision in specialized topics or techniques. Like DC/TMH, distance supervision can be conducted via multiple modalities, including telephone or videoconferencing, or via supervision platforms (Deane et al., 2015). Distance supervision can be used to supervise individuals engaging in DC/TMH or F2F services. As discussed, deliberate practice allows a counselor to practice skills via audio or video recording and transmit them to a supervisor (Elliot et al., 2018; Fredrickson & Rousmaniere, 2018). Following the COVID-19 crisis, several supervisors converted to online supervision, either via telephone or videoconferencing. Like counselors, these supervisors may not have had training in distance supervision, such as the supervision program offered through the Online Therapy Institute. Previously, distance supervision was included in some of the Distance Credentialed Counselor training programs, but is not currently listed as one of the nine content areas required for the BC-TMH training.

Distance supervision, like DC/TMH, must be practiced with caution. Both the supervisor and the supervisee should be trained in distance technologies (Coursol et al., 2016). The supervisor's gatekeeping responsibilities will be challenged by the distance between supervisor and supervisee, specifically if nonverbal cues are reduced during supervision. While the use of "share screen features" allows counselors to share recordings of their sessions, counselors must ensure that their systems meet all HIPAA confidentiality and encryption requirements. Similarly, counselors that send files to supervisors must do so only via secure technology. Many supervisors use small group or triadic supervision. In these circumstances, the supervisor is required to establish guidelines that prohibit taping or recording of supervision sessions which may contain videos on client sessions. Videoconferencing technology allows the option for "remove live" supervision (Fredrickson & Rousmaniere, 2018, p. 183), which is similar to live supervision where a supervisor observes a client/counselor interaction and provides prompts to the counselor through a bug-in-the-ear device. Through remote live supervision, the supervisor "joins" the counseling session without a camera or microphone but is able to observe the client/counselor videoconference session. The supervisor is able to provide prompts and feedback to the counselor, which are only visible to the counselor, via the chat feature in these system (Fredrickson & Rousmaniere, 2018). Sykes Stretch et al. (2016) provide a framework for technology in supervision, including concepts such as legal and ethical guidelines, informed consent, supervisor qualifications, technological issues, security, encryption, confidentiality, record keeping, gatekeeping, and other supervisor requirements.

FUTURE TRENDS IN DISTANCE COUNSELING/TELEMENTAL HEALTH COUNSELING

The future is unknown, and in many ways, so is the future of DC. On average, human beings often don't know, or can't predict, what technology they may want or need in the future. If you had asked someone in 1985 if they needed a computer in their home, they likely would have said no. If you asked someone in 1990 if they needed a mobile phone, they may have scoffed. Even when people know technology exists for others, they often don't see a need for themselves to utilize that technology. More recent technologies, such as music streaming, video streaming, cloud storage, and digital payments, take time to become commonplace, and it is difficult to predict the tipping point at which these technologies become the norm, and everything else is obsolete. So what about DC/TMH counseling?

It is unlikely that F2F counseling will become obsolete. Counselors may fear that technology will replace the human interactions that are essential to professional counseling. Part of this fear may come from the misunderstanding that technology will be used to replace counseling, as opposed to supporting, supplementing, and expanding counseling. "Ideas and practices that are held dear, that work effectively and with which [counselors] are both comfortable and confident, suddenly are confronted with competing alternatives that promise to be faster, more accurate and cheaper" (Bright, 2015, p. 27). However, foundations of human development and psychology dictate that the need for human connection is essential to psychological and interpersonal well-being. Maslow's hierarchy of needs (1943) indicates that beyond physiological needs and safety needs, humans have a need for love and belongingness which includes intimate relationships, family, friends, and social relationships. Furthermore, counseling and psychotherapy have been labeled the talking cure by Freud and colleagues, indicating the therapeutic value that is provided through talking, awareness of nonverbal body language, and even periods of silence between counselor and client (Marx et al., 2017). So while the foundational need for human interaction is unlikely to change, what will likely change are the ways in which we experience these interactions.

Counseling via distance modalities, such as telephone, video conferencing, text, email and chat, have been addressed throughout this book, as well as brief discussions on other modalities, such as mobile apps and Internet-based cognitive behavioral therapy (iCBT). It is expected that new technologies will emerge, beyond technologies currently being used. The use of mobile applications ("apps") will grow in support of either F2F or DC/TMH interventions. Mobile apps already have the capacity to provide real-time data on client symptomology via client self-report. As discussed, these data can provide a more accurate assessment of client functioning, as compared to client recall in weekly sessions. Currently apps are used to walk clients through CBT and mindfulness interventions, provide medication reminders, and connect clients to emergency and recovery resources. Proactive mobile apps are beginning to emerge that will be able to alert the client of a possible mental health concern, as opposed to the client referencing the app when they become aware of symptoms. Zimmerman and Magnavita (2018) describe technologies that use voice recognition software to detect speech patterns indicative of mania or depression, which then alert the individual that an intervention may be needed. Similarly, the professional will likely experience an increase in the use of mental health wearable technologies, which are devices that monitor biological functioning in relation to emotional well-being. Wearable technologies have been utilized by criminal justice systems to monitor blood alcohol content through one's skin for persons under court supervision. These technologies can also be used to monitor issues such as medication compliance or physical symp-toms, such as increased heart rates that may signify anxiety. Like proactive mobile apps, these technologies can either signal the wearer that they may be in need of a mental health intervention, or provide data to mental health providers on client functioning. Concepts such as artificial intelligence (AI) and virtual reality (VR) already impact DC/TMH counseling. It has been discussed how AI and VR interventions can be utilized to improve training of professional counselors, and help counselors practice respond-ing to crises or unstable scenarios. There will likely be an increase in clini-cal interventions utilizing VR, similar to the current use of VR Prolonged Exposure Therapy used to treat posttraumatic stress disorder (PTSD) and phobias (Kothgassner et al., 2019).

Internet self-help is already being widely used for mental health concerns. This trend will continue to grow, particularly as more people have access to creating their own web-based information. Along with this growth comes ethical responsibility for counselors creating or recom-mending self-help resources. One of the challenges of Internet-guided self-help (IGSH) is that IGSH may not be fully encompassed under current ethical codes and guidelines. This book has addressed multiple counseling codes in relation to DC/TMH content, yet much of that content focuses on client/counselor interactions as opposed to IGSH (Borgueta et al., 2017). Ethical guidelines for IGSH may be difficult to manage in the absence of a professional association's ethical guidance (Stricker, 2018). Develop-ers have a responsibility to determine if a program is designed to pro-vide guidance or therapy, as well as a responsibility to manage clinical risk (Borgueta et al., 2017). Additionally, while counselors are encouraged to utilized technology for entrepreneurial opportunities, counselors are equally cautioned to ensure that empirically-based psychological concepts and client well-being are at the center of these initiatives. Counselors are cautioned to avoid developers "whose primary allegiance is toward profit and not necessarily patient care" (Sobelman & Magnavita, 2018, p. 195). Finally, counselors who recommend apps or IGSH have a responsibility to ensure that the tool is appropriate for the clients they serve, and avoids the potential for harm. In an evaluation of mental health mobile apps, researchers found that mobile app messaging and marketing implied that mental health disorders were normal, but also that the responsibility for managing one's mental health was on the individual, as opposed to seek-ing outside assistance. Of greater concern, researchers found that apps framed mental health concerns for those who are white, employed, and part of a family, and failed to acknowledge external or societal stressors that marginalized populations experience (Parker et al., 2018).

The use of technology will continue to grow and expand within the field of counseling, whether practicing in F2F or DC/TMH modali-ties. This book has attempted to emphasize the counselor's role in using technology equitably and effectively among the populations they serve. While DC/TMH interventions are becoming well-known in the counseling and helping professions, consumer awareness may be low. Clients and students may be unaware that DC/TMH interventions are an option, or may be unaware of how to identify a qualified and competent DC/TMH provider. The future of DC/TMH counseling will need to include a public awareness campaign on the risks, benefits, and accessibility of DC/TMH interventions, including issues of limited access for some populations due to cultural, geographic, socioeconomic, or medical coverage differences. A public awareness campaign will require consistency from the counseling profession in relation to training and certification requirements, as well as ethical practice. The challenges of consistency in DC/TMH training and certification have been belabored in this book. While most ethical codes include DC/TMH practices, the use of mobile apps and self-help resources are not well addressed. Counselors will need to advocate for ethical practice and equitable access in their use of DC/TMH interventions, possibly for years to come.

CONCLUSION

The use of DC/TMH interventions in professional counseling will continue to play a primary role in professional counseling for the foreseeable future. As DC/TMH interventions persist, the counseling profession will continue to struggle with the need to require DC/TMH training and certification, or the need to implement DC/TMH instructional practice in counselor education programs. Similarly, licensure laws, regulations, and insurance providers will need to determine the necessity of standardized DC/TMH training. National certifications, such as the BC-TMH, don't currently allow for nonclinical counselor certification. Regardless, the speed at which technology advances requires counselors who utilize DC/TMH interventions to remain current in their knowledge and training through continuing education. A multitude of options for professional development include webinars, online courses, virtual conferences, and deliberate practice. A variety of resources are available to the public to increase their understanding of DC/TMH interventions.

Those considering DC/TMH practice are urged to engage in a variety of self-reflection and planning activities prior to implementation. Additionally, like all professional counselors, counselors utilizing DC/TMH interventions are urged to engage in active self-care, specifically as boundaries may be blurred through TMH interventions. Counselors utilize TMH to assist clients in crisis, which in turn may increase their propensity for burnout and vicarious trauma, as well as feelings of helplessness in relation to social justice and inequity issues. Strategies to avoid burnout include setting boundaries and developing self-compassion. Counselor educators and supervisors will also utilize DC/TMH interventions and must monitor trainees for burnout. Future counseling trends will include increased usage of mobile applications and IGSH, as well as virtual reality, AI, and wearable technologies. These advances and expanded practices will require ethical competence, and equitable use among DC/TMH counselors and the clients they serve.

REFERENCES

American Counseling Association. (2014). *2014 ACA code of ethics.* https://www .counseling.org/Resources/aca-code-of-ethics.pdf

American Telemedicine Association. (2020). *Resources.* https://www.american telemed.org/resource

Borgueta, A. M., Purvis, C. K., & Newman, M. G. (2017). Navigating the ethics of Internet-guided self-help interventions. *Clinical Psychology Science and Practice, 25*, 1–11. https://doi.org/10.1111/cpsp.12235

Bright, J. (2015). If you go down to the woods today, you are in for a big surprise: Seeing the wood for the trees in online delivery of career guidance. *British Journal of Guidance & Counselling, 43*, 24–35. https://doi.org/10.1080/03069885 .2014.979760

Bureau of Labor Statistics. (2020). *The employment situation.* https://www.bls.gov/ news.release/pdf/empsit.pdf

Center for Credentialing in Education. (2020). *Board-Certified-Telemental Health Provider (BC-TMH).* https://www.cce-global.org/credentialing/bctmh

Centers for Disease Control and Prevention. (2020). *COVID-19 in racial and ethnic minority groups.* https://www.cdc.gov/coronavirus/2019-ncov/need-extra -precautions/racial-ethnic-minorities.html

Coaston, S. C. (2017). Self-care through self-compassion: A balm for burn out. *The Professional Counselor, 7*, 285–297. https://doi.org/10.15241/scc.7.3.285

Cooper, L., Briggs, L., & Bagshaw, S. (2018). Postdisaster counselling: Personal, professional, and ethical issues. *Australian Social Work, 4*, 430–443. https://doi .org/10.1080/0312407X.2018.1492622

Council on the Accreditation of Counseling and Related Education Programs. (2016). *2016 CACREP Standards and Glossary.* http://www.cacrep.org/ wp-content/uploads/2018/05/2016-Standards-with-Glossary-5.3.2018.pdf

Coursol, D. N., Lewis, J., & Seymour, J. W. (2016). Cybersupervision: Supervision in a technological age. In S. Goss, K. Anthony, L. Sykes Stretch, & D. Merz Nagel (Eds.), *Technology in mental health: Applications in practice, supervision, and training.* Charles C. Thomas Publishers.

Deane, F. P., Gonsalvez, C., Blackman, R., Saffiotti, D., & Andresen, R. (2015). Issues in the development of e-supervision in professional psychology: A review. *Australian Psychological Society, 50*, 241–247. https://doi.org/10.1111/ap.12107

Elliot, J., Abbass, A., & Rousmaniere, T. (2018). Technology-assisted deliberate practice for improving psychotherapy effectiveness. In J. J. Magnavita (Ed.), *Using technology in mental health practice*. American Psychological Association.

Epstein Becker Green Law. (2017). *50-state survey of telemental/telebehavioral health. (2017 Appendix)*. https://www.ebglaw.com/content/uploads/2017/10/EPSTEIN-BECKER-GREEN-2017-APPENDIX-50-STATE-TELEMENTAL-HEALTH-SURVEY.pdf

Fredrickson, J., & Rousmaniere, T. (2018). Using technology for therapist self-development. In J. J. Magnavita (Ed.), *Using technology in mental health practice*. American Psychological Association.

Gerig, M. S. (2018). *Foundations for clinical mental health counseling: An introduction to the profession* (3rd ed.). Pearson.

Kothgassner, O. D., Goreis, A., Kafka, J. K., Van Eickels, R., L., Plener, P. L., & Felnhofer, A. (2019). Virtual reality exposure therapy for posttraumatic stress disorder (PTSD): a meta-analysis. *European Journal of Psychotraumatology, 10*(1), 1654782. https://doi.org/10.1080/20008198.2019.1654782

Lindo, N. A., Meany Walen, K. K., Ceballos, P., Ohrt, J., Prosek, E., Yousef, D., Yaites, L., Ener, E., & Blalock, S. (2015). Wellness and burnout prevention: Perceptions of a group supervision intervention. *Journal of Professional Counseling: Practice, Theory, and Research, 42*, 28–42. https://doi.org/10.1080/15566382.2015.12033947

Marx, C., Benecke, C., & Gumz, A. (2017). Talking cure models: A framework of analysis. *Frontiers in Psychology, 8*, 1–13. https://doi.org/10.3389/fpsyg.2017.01589

Maslow, A. H. (1943). A theory of human motivation. *Psychological Review, 50*(4), 370–396. https://doi.org/10.1037/h0054346

Master's in Psychology and Counseling Accreditation Council. (2017). *Accreditation manual*. http://mpcacaccreditation.org/wp-content/uploads/2020/05/MPCAC2017AccreditationManual050520.pdf

Naghavi, A., & Salimi, S. (2018). An autoethnography of vicarious trauma and vicarious growth in the context of rehabilitation counseling. *Iran Journal of Psychiatric Behavioral Sciences, 12*, 1–6. https://doi.org/10.5812/ijpbs.62687

Nelson, J. R., Hall, B. S., Anderson, J. L., Birtles, C., & Hemming, L. (2018). Self-compassion as self-care: A simple and effective tool for counselor educators and counseling students. *Journal of Creativity in Mental Health, 13*, 121–133. https://doi.org/10.1080/15401383.2017.1328292

New York State Office of Mental Health. (2020). *Mental health resources during an emergency*. https://omh.ny.gov/omhweb/disaster_resources/pandemic_influenza

Online Therapy Institute. (2020). *For therapists*. https://www.onlinetherapyinstitute.com/therapists

Parker, L., Bero, L., Gillies, D., Raven, M., Mintez, B., Jureidini, J., & Grundy, Q. (2018). Mental health messages in prominent mental health apps. *Annals of Family Medicine, 8*(16), 338–342. https://doi.org/10.1370/afm.2260

Remley, T. P., & Herlihy, B. (2016). *Ethical, legal, and professional issues in counseling.* Pearson.

Riva, G., & Repetto, C. (2016). Using virtual reality immersion therapeutically. In S. Goss, K. Anthony, L. Sykes Stretch, & D. Merz Nagel (Eds.), *Technology in mental health: Applications in practice, supervision, and training.* Charles C. Thomas Publishers.

Roysircar, G. (2009). The big picture of advocacy: Counselor, heal society and thyself. *Journal of Counseling and Development, 87,* 288–294. https://doi .org/10.1002/j.1556-6678.2009.tb00109.x

Sobelman, S. A., & Magnavita, J. J. (2018). Extending your mental health practice as an entrepreneur. In J. J. Magnavita (Ed.), *Using technology in mental health practice.* American Psychological Association.

Stricker, G. (2018). Ethical considerations for internet-guides self-help interventions. *Clinical Psychological Science and Practice, 25,* e12240. https://doi.org/10.1111/ cpsp.12240

Substance Abuse and Mental Health Services Administration. (2020, April 22). *CCBHCs using telehealth or telemedicine.* https://www.samhsa.gov/section-223/ care-coordination/telehealth-telemedicine

Sykes Stretch, L., Merz Nagel, D., & Anthony, K. (2016). An updated ethical framework for the use of technology in supervision. In S. Goss, K. Anthony, L. Sykes Stretch, & D. Merz Nagel (Eds.), *Technology in mental health: Applications in practice, supervision, and training.* Charles C. Thomas Publishers.

World Health Organization. (2020, April 28). *Coronavirus disease 2019 (COVID-19) Situation report-99.* https://www.who.int/docs/default-source/coronaviruse/ situation-reports/20200428-sitrep-99-covid-19.pdf?sfvrsn=119fc381_2

Zimmerman, J., & Magnavita, J. J. (2018). Adapting new technology for your practice: How to assess fit and risks. In J. J. Magnavita (Ed.), *Using technology in mental health practice.* American Psychological Association.

Zur Institute. (2020). *Digital ethics, HIPAA, and telemental health.* https://www .zurinstitute.com/resources/hipaa/#telemental_health_top

Appendix 12.A

CHECKLIST OF DISTANCE COUNSELING/TELEMENTAL HEALTH PRACTICE

This checklist is designed to provide the reader with foundational tasks required in establishing a DC/TMH practice, or reflecting on a practice already established. For each item, readers are asked to indicate if they have completed that task ("Yes"), or if they have not or are unsure ("No/ Unsure"). The checklist also includes a column for "Date Achieved or Deadline" where readers are expected to enter the date at which they achieved the items entered or plan to achieve them. These 55 tasks have been addressed throughout the book and readers are encouraged to review relevant items and chapters as they plan for their practice. Each item is an opportunity for reflection, decision-making, and preparation. The goal is that these items will be achieved and documented as you prepare for your practice.

The checklist is divided by Preparation for Practice, Logistics of Practice, and Engaging in Practice, however all elements of the checklist should be reviewed and achieved prior to practice. Minimally, counselors should be reflecting on these items and how they would address them in their professional practice, in order to be prepared for circumstances as they arise. *Finally, this checklist is presented as a general guideline. It is not exhaustive and it is not definitive. It is designed as a starting point for professional practice, and does not include elements of counseling specializations and specific circumstances.*

PREPARATION FOR PRACTICE	YES	NO OR UNSURE	DATE ACHIEVED OR DEADLINE
1. Are you aware of both the evidence-based effectiveness and professional limitations of DC and TMH services?			

(continued)

PREPARATION FOR PRACTICE	YES	NO OR UNSURE	DATE ACHIEVED OR DEADLINE
2. Are you able to explain both the evidence-based effectiveness and professional limitations of DC/TMH services to your clients/students and potential clients/students?			
3. Are you aware of the laws in your state and jurisdiction pertaining to DC/TMH practice? Did you confirm this information with the state or jurisdiction?			
4. Are you aware of geographic limitations pertaining to your DC/TMH practice?			
5. If your specialization does not require state license, do you know what your profession or national certification indicates about distance practice?			
6. Do you have training or certification in DC/TMH? If not, do you know how you can obtain it prior to practice?			
7. Does your malpractice insurance cover you for DC/TMH practice? If applicable, do your insurance panels cover DC/TMH?			
8. Do you know what modality you plan to use to practice DC/TMH; e.g., telephone, videoconference, email?			
9. Are you technologically competent to effectively utilize the technology for your planned DC/TMH interventions?			
10. Will you offer planned DC/TMH services?			
11. Will you provide synchronous DC/TMH services?			
12. Will you provide asynchronous DC/TMH services?			
13. Will you use a blended platform?			
14. Will you use a turnkey platform?			
15. Do you have verification that all technology you will use is secure, encrypted, HIPAA compliant, and able to protect ePHI? Consider phone, email, record keeping, and all technology used in your practice.			

(continued)

PREPARATION FOR PRACTICE	YES	NO OR UNSURE	DATE ACHIEVED OR DEADLINE
16. If you are using a third-party software or vendors, did you obtain a business associate agreement from each provider?			
17. Have you thoroughly reviewed the entirety of ethical codes for your professional counseling organization, as well as related organizations, including content on DC/TMH practice?			
18. Have you created a detailed informed consent document, pertaining to planned and unplanned DC/TMH services?			
19. Does your DC/TMH informed consent document include all items required from your code of ethics, including risks and benefits of TMH, anticipated response times, and others?			
20. Does your informed consent document include a detailed safety plan, including the ability to manage crises from a distance?			
21. Does your informed consent document include a counselor-not-available contact plan?			
22. Does your informed consent document include a plan for verifying client identity?			
23. Do you have a detailed social media policy which you review with all clients equally?			
24. Are you willing to create separate social media accounts for personal and professional use?			
25. Do you have a policy for voice-assisted technologies that you review with all clients equally?			
26. Have you assessed if DC/TMH interventions are appropriate for the population you serve (e.g., developmentally, clinically, culturally)?			
27. Have you assessed if the clients/students you serve have equitable access to technology?			
28. Have you assessed your clients'/students' preference to receive DC/TMH interventions, as opposed to F2F services?			

(continued)

PREPARATION FOR PRACTICE	YES	NO OR UNSURE	DATE ACHIEVED OR DEADLINE
29. Have you assessed your own cultural competence and ability to work with diverse populations via DC/TMH interventions?			
30. Have you identified resources to support your practice including professional organizations and supervision, including peer supervisors who are experienced with DC/TMH use?			

LOGISTICS OF PRACTICE	YES	NO OR UNSURE	DATE ACHIEVED OR DEADLINE
31. Do you have access to a professional workspace, free from distractions, where you are able to maintain privacy and client confidentiality?			
32. Do you have a plan to manage distractions or privacy concerns in relation to your clients'/students' setting?			
33. Do you have a plan for protecting client privacy and confidentiality, both in relation to session content and maintaining records?			
34. Do you have a plan to verify client location at the beginning of each session, and cross reference that location with safety plan content?			
35. Do you have secure reliable technology that will minimize the opportunity for technological breakdowns and slowdowns?			
36. Do you have a plan for technology disruptions in your informed consent document?			
37. Do you have access to wired Internet and phone service if needed?			
38. If you use a professional website, is the website up to date with reputable information, and is accessible to diverse populations?			
39. Do you have a complaint procedure posted on your website or in your informed consent document, including links to professional licensing board or organizations?			
40. Do you have a plan to update your technology regularly?			

(continued)

LOGISTICS OF PRACTICE	YES	NO OR UNSURE	DATE ACHIEVED OR DEADLINE
41. If you provide referrals to websites, mobile apps, or self-help services, are you verifying that those resources are accurate, evidence-based, and reputable?			
42. Do you have a process for securing client records, along with a plan to dispose of client records appropriately?			
43. Are you using secure and encrypted email to send information, or another secure mechanism to send/receive client information?			
44. Do you have a plan to manage referrals to F2F services or other counseling specializations, particularly when the client is out of your geographic region?			
45. Do you have a plan to screen clients prior to services, including group and individual clients, to assess their appropriateness for DC/TMH interventions?			

ENGAGING IN PRACTICE	YES	NO OR UNSURE	DATE ACHIEVED OR DEADLINE
46. Do you have the knowledge and skills to maintain and enhance the client-counselor relationship while using DC/TMH interventions?			
47. If you are using videoconferencing, are you aware of appropriate distances and background images for professional counseling?			
48. If you are using videoconferencing, are you aware of how to improve eye contact and how to explain variations in eye contact to your clients/students?			
49. Do you know how to identify emotions in clients and how you may need to alter these practices using DC/TMH interventions?			
50. Do you have a plan to manage a potential lack of nonverbal communication, as well as silence, during DC/TMH sessions?			

(continued)

ENGAGING IN PRACTICE	YES	NO OR UNSURE	DATE ACHIEVED OR DEADLINE
51. If you will engage in group work, do you know which modality you will utilize; e.g., telephone, videoconferencing, discussion boards?			
52. If you will engage in group work, have you established group rules for your DC/TMH group?			
53. If you will engage in group work, do you have a plan to manage talk time and silence?			
54. Do you have a plan to manage DC/TMH group dynamics, including engaging clients, managing monopolizers, and controlling cross-talk?			
55. Most importantly, whether facilitating individual or group DC/TMH session, do you have a plan for managing clients in crisis, including upholding your duty to warn?			

Index

Printed in the USA
CPSIA information can be obtained
at www.ICGtesting.com
CBHW072324041224
18471CB00005B/178

9 780826 179944